Prostate Cancer

A FAMILY CONSULTATION

Prostate Cancer

A Family Consultation

Philip Kantoff, M.D.
with Malcolm McConnell

HOUGHTON MIFFLIN COMPANY

BOSTON • NEW YORK   1996

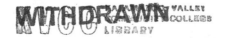

Library of Congress Cataloging-in-Publication Data
Kantoff, Philip
    Prostate cancer : a family consultation / Philip Kantoff,
with Malcolm McConnell.
        p.   cm.
    Includes bibliographical references and index.
    ISBN 0-395-84549-1
    ISBN 0-395-71823-6 (pbk.)
    1. Prostate — Cancer — Popular works. I. McConnell,
Malcolm. II. Title.
RC280.P7K36   1996   96-22152
616.99'463 — dc20   CIP

Printed in the United States of America

Book design by Robert Overholtzer

QUM 10 9 8 7 6 5 4 3 2 1

The names of the persons mentioned in the case
histories have been altered to protect their privacy.

Contents

This book is dedicated to my wife, Rochelle, my children, Aaron, Emily, and Sydney, my parents, Lisa and Sidney, and my sister, Gwen, who all have been my inspiration. I am also indebted to my patients, who have entrusted me with their care and from whom I have learned so much.

Introduction

I am a medical oncologist who specializes in treating men with prostate cancer. As the director of genitourinary oncology at the Dana-Farber Cancer Institute in Boston, I coordinate patient care and research related to this illness. I also teach and conduct research at Harvard Medical School.

I spend a great deal of time consulting with men who have been diagnosed with the disease. Since I do not perform surgery or administer radiation therapy, the two principal forms of treatment for early stages of prostate cancer, you can consider me a neutral referee, a physician who represents patients' interests and offers the perspective of medical science as you and your family consider which treatments are best for you.

Choosing among prostate cancer treatment options can be a confusing and frightening decision. The cause of the fear is obvious: any cancer is terrifying. However, you can often be cured of prostate cancer if it is detected and treated in its early stage. The confusion about your risk of developing prostate cancer, your need to be screened, and, if diagnosed with the disease, what treatment is best for you, springs from several roots.

First, for both patients and physicians, the perception of prostate cancer has changed dramatically in the past ten years, due primarily to the increasing numbers of men now being diagnosed. Ten years ago, if you thought about prostate cancer at all, you probably considered it an obscure affliction of very old men. But today, you are regularly hammered by television and newspaper stories about the "epidemic" of prostate cancer that is sweeping the country. Indeed, prostate cancer is now the most commonly diagnosed cancer in America, with 317,000 cases and 41,400 deaths expected in 1996. Recently, the number of men each year who had radical prostatectomies — surgical procedures to remove their cancerous prostates — rose to over 100,000.

Naturally you ask, *is* there really a prostate cancer epidemic? The answer is no. But how does this apparent explosion of prostate cancer cases in recent years affect you and your family? Are you more at risk of dying from prostate cancer today than your father was twenty or thirty years ago?

Again, the answer is encouraging. The increased risk of death is extremely small. But there is certainly a dramatic rise in diagnosed prostate cancer cases, due largely to two unrelated factors: the increased number of men potentially susceptible to the disease as our population ages, and the markedly improved ability to detect prostate cancer, mostly due to the development and widespread use of the Prostate Specific Antigen (PSA) test.

The postwar baby boom generation, the largest population cohort in American history, is now firmly entrenched in middle age: almost 4 million men turn 50 each year. The health consciousness of today's middle-aged Americans has reduced the number of deaths caused by the traditional principal killer, cardiovascular disease. American men are living longer, and thus ironically are having a greater chance of being diagnosed with prostate cancer.

The PSA test, a relatively recent medical innovation, has incorrectly been described as a blood test for prostate cancer. The test measures the level of a protein secreted by only the prostate gland. High levels of PSA are suggestive — but not diagnostic proof — of prostate cancer. A patient with an elevated PSA often will need to undergo a biopsy of the prostate. The improved method of taking biopsy samples involves the use of a spring-loaded needle gun that is precisely guided by an ultrasound probe. This technique, which is more accurate and causes fewer side effects than the older method, has increased the prostate cancer detection rates. Because more men today are routinely receiving the PSA test and biopsies, cancer is being detected at earlier stages.

News stories, however, often make it seem as if prostate cancer is spreading unchecked through the ranks of middle-aged and elderly American men. This has created confusion and fear among millions of Americans, sparking discussions in both the lay press and professional journals over what to tell the public about this important *new* health problem.

Unfortunately, we haven't educated American men and their families well about prostate cancer. Medical experts often have opposing viewpoints on almost every aspect of prostate cancer, from screening and diagnosis to treatment options for early cancer to the management of more advanced stages of the disease. For example, the medical profession remains uncertain about the impact PSA screening and subsequent treatment have on the most important issues, such as survival rate and quality of life. You don't want to be enmeshed in this medical debate — you want clear answers to your questions. My goal is to provide you with answers.

Screening and treatment of prostate cancer may help hundreds of thousands of men. But you should know that medical intervention can have a negative impact on you and your family. You may be among the men who suffer emotional and physical pain as you are swept away in the screening and treatment processes. In recent years I have seen a disturbing pattern among the men who come to me for consultation. Often they are caught in a rapid and confusing chain of events that leaves them vulnerable.

During a routine physical exam, a man undergoes the Prostate Specific Antigen test, which detects an elevated level of PSA. A biopsy is then taken, which may reveal early, potentially curable prostate cancer. X-rays and other scans may be ordered over the ensuing week or two. The next step would be a return visit to the urologist, when the doctor states, "I've scheduled you for surgery in two weeks." The message is clear: the patient has cancer, and the sooner the malignancy is removed the better.

Many of the strong advocates of increased awareness and treatment of prostate cancer are men who were diagnosed with the disease, received treatment, and are now survivors. We've read the accounts of Bob Dole, Norman Schwarzkopf, and Jerry Lewis, who owe their lives to rapid diagnosis and treatment. But the number of men who have recently died from prostate cancer makes us worry about the "epidemic." The victims include François Mitterrand, Steve Ross of Time-Warner, Frank Zappa, and Telly Savalas. The controversial millionaire Michael Milken, whose advanced prostate cancer is in remission, may be the most active advocate of increased public awareness and research.

However, sufficient scientific information is not yet available to help you, your family, and your physician determine which diagnosis and treatment options are most appropriate. Oversimplified accounts hailing the PSA test as an early diagnosis tool that is equivalent to mammogram screening for breast cancer don't help clarify this confusion; nor do stories that imply few prostate cancer patients actually need to be treated at all (watchful waiting is the preferred therapy option in Europe). You should carefully consider all of the prostate cancer treatment options before deciding which is best for you. Don't be pressured into quickly accepting one particular form of treatment until all your other options have been carefully weighed.

The only way to prove with scientific certainty the benefit of a particular prostate cancer treatment is with research. However, the questions my colleagues are addressing today about the value of different treatment options won't provide us with detailed information for several years.

What should you do while waiting for these research findings? Educate yourself as well as possible about the nature of the disease, your likelihood of being diagnosed with it, and what treatments are best for your individual needs. In other words, plan a thorough consultation with a medical specialist in prostate cancer.

In the chapters that follow, I will provide you a detailed and compassionate consultation much as I do every day with my patients.

I consider the time I spend describing the benefits and risks of treatment options an excellent investment in my patients' future. Making a decision with adequate information lessens their fear and uncertainty and helps guide them and their families to an appropriate treatment. But I also realize that the thousands of people I have advised and treated represent only a tiny fraction of the hundreds of thousands of Americans — many in the prime of their productive lives — who each year hear the frightening words "You have prostate cancer."

In a face-to-face consultation, there is a great deal of give and take between my patients and me. They and their families ask questions, and I reply in as much detail as possible. Although we can't follow this pattern in a book, I do try to retain as much of the consultation format as possible.

Approaching this book as I would an office consultation, I often address you, the reader, as "you." Obviously, you do not fit every case pattern in my description of screening, diagnosis, treatment options (including surgery and radiation therapy), their cure potential, their side effects, and the advanced course of the disease. But since this book is a thorough consultation and it is vital for you to learn as much as you can about prostate cancer if you are to make the appropriate decisions, please read the book from beginning to end, building on the information I present in a logical sequence to gain a full understanding of the impact prostate cancer may have on your life.

I begin by describing the prostate gland in its noncancerous condition. Then I explain the nature of prostate cancer and how the diagnosis is made through the screening and biopsy process. I go on to discuss treatment options for local disease (meaning the tumor is confined to the gland), addressing cure potential and side effects.

For men who have more advanced disease — cancer that has escaped the confines of the gland — I carefully explain the disease progression and the extensive range of treatments we now have available. Men with either localized or advanced disease should take advantage of the well-established prostate cancer patient-support groups that now exist in almost every American city. I hope that this format is as helpful to you and your family as it is to my patients.

I include lists of questions people commonly ask during consultations about the different phases of the disease and its treatment. If you or a loved one develops prostate cancer, do ask these questions when you see your physicians.

During consultations, I follow certain principles. I firmly believe that my patients and I must be equal partners, striving to make the best possible decisions on a case-by-case basis. The critical questions we address as partners include:

- Should I be screened with the Prostate Specific Antigen test?
- If I have an elevated PSA level, what further diagnostic steps should I take?
- If the evaluation reveals prostate cancer, should I be treated?
- What form of treatment is best for me? How will treatment affect the quality of my life?
- What are the options open to me if it is discovered that I already have advanced disease?

These questions are deceptively simple. It is my primary professional responsibility to help you answer them, and there is a complex set of factors that must be considered as we weigh these options.

Keep in mind that I am committed to form the same type of partnership with you that I do with my patients in guiding them through a confusing and frightening period of their lives. So I consider this book to be a natural extension of my joint roles of physician, researcher, and teacher.

1

The Prostate Gland: Noncancerous Conditions of the Prostate

The Prostate Gland

If you are like many men, you may not even know where your prostate gland is located. The prostate surrounds the urethra between the base of the bladder and the muscular sheet that makes up the floor of the pelvic cavity. The prostate is nestled at the bottom of this cavity, surrounded by blood vessels, nerves, and connective tissue. All male mammals have some type of a prostate gland; it is fundamental to our evolution.

The primary function of the prostate gland is to produce semen. Semen consists of proteins and other chemicals that nourish the sperm and are critical to male fertility. The portion of the semen made in the prostate helps preserve and transport the sperm that are formed in the testicles and stored in the adjacent epididymis. Without the prostate, reproduction through sexual intercourse would be impossible.

Anatomy of the Prostate

The principal components of the male reproductive system — the testicles (with the epididymis and vas deferens), the seminal vesicles, the prostate, and the penis — must all function in close

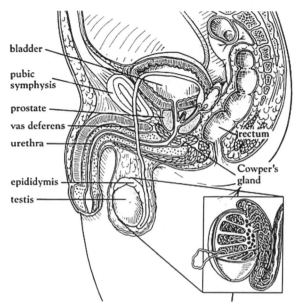

bladder

pubic
symphysis

prostate

vas deferens

urethra

epididymis

testis

rectum

Cowper's
gland

1. Anatomy of the male reproductive system
(Courtesy, Merck Human Health Division)

coordination for successful ejaculation. Spermatozoa are produced by cells in the testes and become mature sperm within the
tightly coiled tubes of the epididymis, which are located on the
head of each testis.

At the time of orgasm, when ejaculation occurs, the sperm are
expelled through two long muscular tubes called the vas deferens,
which we commonly call the vas. The two vas pass beside the pair
of seminal vesicles; the four structures meet at the ejaculatory
duct within the prostatic urethra. Here the prostatic fluid joins
the mixture of semen from the vas and seminal vesicles. The fluid
is expelled through the urethra by powerful muscle contractions
(*see figure 3*). You can think of the prostate as secreting the complex mix of supporting chemicals; the testicles make the actual
sperm. The testicles, prostate, and adjacent seminal vesicles must
work in unison to produce viable semen (*see figure 1*).

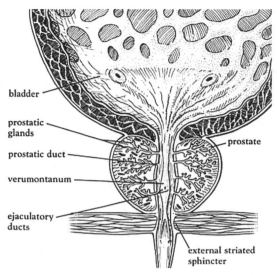

2. The prostate and surrounding structures
(Courtesy, Merck Human Health Division)

Women do not have a prostate gland; they have a remnant structure in their pelvis called the Skenes glands. This gland complex is much smaller than the prostate and serves no obvious function at this stage of our evolution, although fluid derived from the gland drains into the female urethra.

An infant's prostate is no larger than a pea. The gland develops to its adult size from exposure to the male hormone testosterone (produced mainly in the testicles), which also brings about other anatomical changes during the maturation process. The adult prostate is a walnut-size gland attached to the bottom of the urinary bladder where it joins the urethra, the tube that runs from the bladder to the exterior of the body through the penis. This small gland surrounds the portion of the urethra adjacent to the bladder. The inner urethral sphincter (one of the muscular valves that controls urine flow) is at the neck of the bladder and at the top of the prostate. The external (striated) urethral sphincter is at the bottom (the apex of the prostate) and is the muscle you use to voluntarily control the flow of urine. The prostate is distinct from the bladder, urethra, and urethral sphincters, although it is in direct contact with these other structures (*see figure 2*).

Your prostate probably measures about an inch and a half wide at its base and slightly less in its vertical diameter, and weighs about twenty grams. The prostate has two sides, which are sometimes referred to as lobes, and the entire structure is covered by a paper-thin capsule. The gland is divided into three zones. The peripheral zone is examined during a digital rectal exam (DRE), the procedure in which a physician inserts a rubber-gloved finger into the rectum to feel the posterior portion of the prostate, checking for swelling, hardness, or irregular nodules that are suggestive of prostate cancer. The prostate's central and transition zones are closer to the urethra (*see figures 3 and 4*).

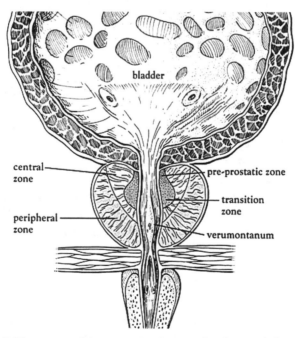

3. The zones of the prostate, cross-section forward view
(Courtesy, Merck Human Health Division)

The prostate is made up of two types of tissue: epithelial (glandular) and connective (stromal). Both types of tissue are unique to the prostate, but only the epithelial tissue produces the prostate-specific antigen detected in the PSA blood test. These glandular cells secrete the chemicals that make up the prostate's contribution to the seminal fluid in a network of hundreds of mini-glands connected by small ducts to the urethra. It is the glandular cells that become cancerous, producing what we know to be prostate cancer.

The stromal or connective tissue component of the prostate is an amorphous fibrous and muscular structure woven around the mini-glands throughout the prostate, thereby supporting the epithelial tissue. Stromal tissue contracts to expel the glandular secretion. The glandular epithelial component is comparable to the pulp of a grapefruit, with the stromal tissue being the fruit's fibrous membrane and the outer capsule its smooth skin (*see figures 5 and 6*).

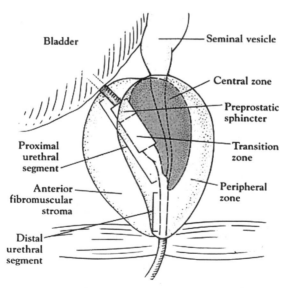

4. The zones of the prostate, cross-section side view
(Courtesy, Merck Human Health Division)

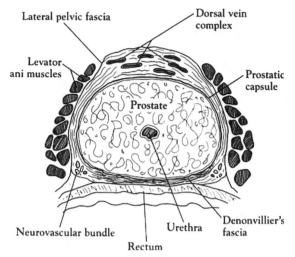

5. The prostate and surrounding structures, cross-section overhead view. Note the position of the neuralvascular bundles and the dorsal vein complex
(Courtesy, Merck Human Health Division)

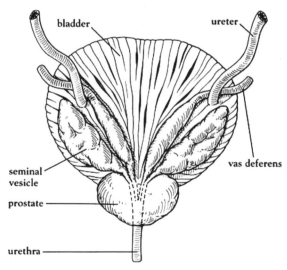

6. The prostate and surrounding structures, posterior view (Courtesy, Merck Human Health Division)

Benign Prostate Conditions

During puberty, increasing levels of male hormones promote the development of the prostate's glandular component. The prostate continues to grow throughout a man's life. At the onset of middle age, the rate of growth in prostate tissue — notably the stromal component — almost always increases. By age 70, the weight of the prostate can average between 30 and 60 grams, compared to 20 grams at age 25.

This enlargement is called benign prostatic hyperplasia (BPH). Due to BPH, the prostate may eventually expand to several times its normal adult volume. The increase in the volume of prostate tissue most frequently involves the stromal tissue, but epithelial tissue can also be involved. The prostate tissue overgrowth of BPH does *not* necessarily result in prostate cancer. BPH and prostate cancer are common and are most likely unrelated. Some men needlessly worry that their BPH will somehow turn into prostate cancer. Many men, however, never even know they have BPH because they're free of symptoms.

Clinical manifestations of BPH, which is sometimes called prostatism, include a diminished urine stream. This results from BPH when the urethra channel through the gland is squeezed and narrowed. BPH may involve your entire prostate, but frequently includes principally that portion of your prostate that encircles the urethra. With the capacity to urinate diminished, your bladder is never adequately emptied. This often results in a nagging urgency to urinate frequently — at times every hour or so — even when the narrowed urethra permits only a dribbling stream. BPH can also lead to frequent urination at night, sometimes even four or more times a night. If the condition becomes severe, the prostatic urethra virtually closes, making urination impossible.

Symptoms of BPH
- Urgency of urination
- Hesitancy during urination

- Frequency of urination
- Frequent urination at nighttime (called nocturia)

If you have these symptoms, you have a problem with your urinary tract. You already may have been diagnosed with BPH. But from my experience as a physician, men have a surprisingly varied tolerance for the discomforts of this condition. Some middle-aged men are alarmed by the first indication that their urine flow is diminished, while many older men accept the interruption of sleep three or four times a night due to the urgency of nocturia. As a general rule, you should tell your physician if you are urinating frequently during the day or more than once in the night. If you do have BPH, ask your physician about the relative severity of your condition.

To better understand BPH and other prostate conditions, including prostate cancer, you should be familiar with the male anatomy.

Prostate tissue surrounding the urethra is called the transition zone. This is where we believe BPH arises, although it may spread to other areas of the prostate. The area that surrounds the transition zone is called the peripheral zone. Most prostate cancers develop in the peripheral zone. Cancers in the posterior peripheral zone can usually be felt in the digital rectal exam: physicians are trained to detect the typical lumpy or gritty texture of prostate cancer by touch. Some cancers arise in the transition zone as well. Most of the cancers that are now being detected through PSA-based screening (PSA test used with DRE) are small tumors in the peripheral zone.

Because I am focusing on prostate cancer in this book, I will not detail the several effective and reliable methods of diagnosis and treatment of BPH now available. If you are experiencing urinary problems, you should see your doctor. Prostate cancer, which may coexist with BPH or occur independently, is most often *not* a cause of symptoms related to urine flow.

Treatment options for BPH include drugs that shrink the prostate or improve the ability of the bladder to empty, and, in more severe cases, surgery to resect or trim the excess BPH tissue. This surgical procedure (transurethral resection of prostate: TURP) involves the use of a cutting device, a laser procedure, or a vaporization procedure by a urologist to remove the enlarged obstructing tissue.

Most urologists view surgery for BPH as a treatment that is best reserved for severe cases or to be undertaken when more conservative medication therapy has failed to relieve symptoms.

Once again, BPH is a benign condition: it is unrelated to the process that takes place during the development of prostate cancer. BPH tissue does not have the potential of spreading to "seed" itself elsewhere in the body, as does a malignant prostate cancer tumor.

Another common condition of the prostate is an inflammation called prostatitis. This is often the result of a bacterial infection and can cause severe discomfort, fever, and chills, as well as pain at the base of the penis or in the rectal area. Prostatitis can be acute — a single episode of varying severity — or chronic, with repeated episodes.

If the condition is bacterial in nature, it is treated with antibiotics. The course of treatment can be longer (up to six weeks) than for other bacterial infections, so don't be alarmed when the doctor prescribes a seemingly long treatment. Prostatitis also can be nonbacterial, and in such cases it is treated with anti-inflammatory medications and warm baths. You are encouraged to eliminate spicy food, alcohol, coffee, and tobacco. Chronic prostatitis presents a more difficult treatment challenge, sometimes requiring antibiotic therapy as well as the measures used for nonbacterial prostatitis.

Keep in mind that, as with BPH, both acute and chronic prostatitis are separate from and do not lead to prostate cancer.

2

Prostate Cancer:
Risk and Prevention

Are You at Risk for Prostate Cancer? If So, How Can You Prevent It?

You probably don't like to think about cancer. If you have avoided even considering your own level of risk for prostate cancer, you're certainly not alone. But the simple fact that you are reading this book means you've reached a point where your natural reluctance to think about cancer has been overcome by a more mature need to educate yourself about the impact of prostate cancer on your life. So, let's start with the basics.

All cancers result from a complex interplay between genetics, or the biological blueprint that we inherit from our parents, and the environment — the substances that we eat, drink, or are otherwise exposed to in our surroundings. Prostate cancer undoubtedly results from some combination of genetic and environmental factors. Although we actually know relatively little about either, some factors are more significant than others.

Age is the single most important factor associated with prostate cancer, since it usually afflicts middle-aged and elderly men. Prostate cancer is extremely rare in men below the age of 40 and very uncommon in men younger than 50. However, the incidence of the disease increases steeply above the age of 50 and is most common for men over 65 (*see table 1, page 15*).

The fact that prostate cancer is a disease associated with advancing age provides hints about its cause and natural history. We

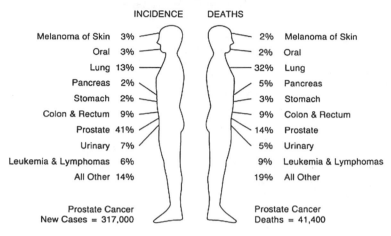

1996 ESTIMATED CANCER INCIDENCE AND MORTALITY
BY SITE FOR MALES

	INCIDENCE			DEATHS	
Melanoma of Skin	3%		2%	Melanoma of Skin
Oral	3%		2%	Oral
Lung	13%		32%	Lung
Pancreas	2%		5%	Pancreas
Stomach	2%		3%	Stomach
Colon & Rectum	9%		9%	Colon & Rectum
Prostate	41%		14%	Prostate
Urinary	7%		5%	Urinary
Leukemia & Lymphomas	6%		9%	Leukemia & Lymphomas
All Other	14%		19%	All Other

Prostate Cancer
New Cases = 317,000

Prostate Cancer
Deaths = 41,400

7. Prostate cancer cases in the United States

do know that the earliest undetected microscopic forms of prostate cancer begin to appear in men in their 30s. Presumably, with the passage of time, the disease becomes "clinically apparent" — it reaches a point where it can be detected by physicians using the DRE or biopsies, for example. But prostate cancer can exist undetected — showing no signs or symptoms — for a number of years, possibly a man's entire life.

There are two explanations for the typically slow progression of prostate cancer. One is that many if not most of the genetic events at the cellular level — mutations — necessary for the creation of prostate cancer probably occur early in life, while it is environmental factors such as diet that allow these microscopic cancers to grow and become dangerous. According to this development theory, we should be able to determine those factors, such as foods, that either inhibit or accentuate the growth of the cancer. An alternative theory is that tiny cancers caused by mutations acquire more and more genetic change over time — possibly independent of the environment — and that microscopic malignancies ultimately, and perhaps inevitably, become large and

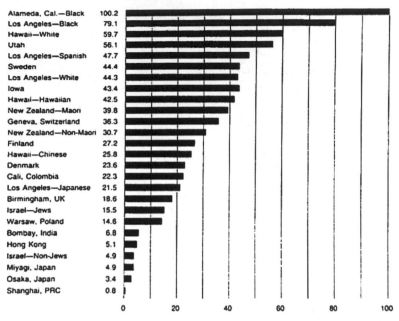

Alameda, Cal.—Black	100.2
Los Angeles—Black	79.1
Hawaii—White	59.7
Utah	56.1
Los Angeles—Spanish	47.7
Sweden	44.4
Los Angeles—White	44.3
Iowa	43.4
Hawaii—Hawaiian	42.5
New Zealand—Maori	39.8
Geneva, Switzerland	36.3
New Zealand—Non-Maori	30.7
Finland	27.2
Hawaii—Chinese	25.8
Denmark	23.6
Cali, Colombia	22.3
Los Angeles—Japanese	21.5
Birmingham, UK	18.6
Israel—Jews	15.5
Warsaw, Poland	14.6
Bombay, India	6.8
Hong Kong	5.1
Israel—Non-Jews	4.9
Miyagi, Japan	4.9
Osaka, Japan	3.4
Shanghai, PRC	0.8

8. Prostate cancer cases worldwide

aggressive cancers. A combination of both of these explanations is most likely valid.

Another feature of prostate cancer is that some groups of men in the world are less likely to acquire the disease, while other populations seem very prone to it. In Asia, particularly in Japan and China, diagnosed prostate cancer is a relatively uncommon disease. But in Scandinavia and the United States, the incidence is relatively high (*see figure 8*).

The incidence of prostate cancer is particularly high among African-American men, with most cases striking inner-city populations. Statistics indicate that African-Americans also have a poorer survival rate for every stage of the disease than white populations. Researchers have not yet determined the extent to which environmental factors such as diet and lifestyle play a role compared to genetic factors. If you are an African-American, you owe it to yourself and your family to keep in mind this increased risk, as well as its particular virulence, as you consider screening and treatment options. Research indicates that when men move from low-incidence areas (such as Japan) to high-incidence areas (such as the United States), their incidence level increases. This suggests that environmental factors are involved.

It is difficult to quantify the role diet plays in the development and progression of prostate cancer, but the food you eat is clearly important. The evidence that dietary fat is important is compelling but is probably a relatively minor factor. Certain types of fat — such as highly saturated animal fat — may be more dangerous than others. My simple advice is to minimize fat intake and increase exercise.

One provocative dietary connection has been made between prostate cancer and tomatoes. My colleagues from the Harvard School of Public Health, led by Ed Giovannucci, have shown that men whose diets were high in tomato-based products developed fewer prostate cancers. You might want to add tomatoes to your diet; this simple dietary adjustment can't hurt, and it just might help decrease your risk of prostate cancer.

Another important aspect of the epidemiology of prostate cancer is that in some cases the disease may be inherited. A gene (the portion of a chromosome that determines a particular trait), or more likely an array of genes, may be passed from parent to child (as we now believe is the pattern with certain types of colon and breast cancer). Research suggests that if several members of your family have been diagnosed with prostate cancer, you have a greater risk of developing the disease. This implies that if a gene or genes are responsible for prostate cancer in a particular family, they will exist in many members of that family. The genetic tendency toward prostate cancer suggests a higher likelihood of multiple family members contracting the disease and the development of the disease at younger ages than normal.

If you see this pattern in your family, however, it does not necessarily mean that the cause of the prostate cancer in your family is the result of an inherited genetic tendency. Nor does this definitely demonstrate that a family with a young prostate cancer victim carries cancer-promoting genes. But the chances that members of such families carry a gene responsible for inherited prostate cancer are increased. So if you have several close blood relatives — especially men younger than 55 — with prostate cancer, you should consider yourself at increased risk.

Even if a small fraction of prostate cancers results from an inherited gene or genes, most prostate tumors arise as a result of more complex and often subtle interplay between your genetics (or cellular blueprint) and the environment. For example, in experiments recently performed in my laboratory at Dana-Farber Cancer Institute, it was determined that different forms of a gene involved with the chemistry of the male hormones called androgens — the androgen receptor gene — influence the likelihood of developing prostate cancer. I think even more importantly, we found that inherited differences in the androgen receptor gene influence the aggressiveness of a cancer, that is, the likelihood that a prostate tumor will be lethal. Testing for this inherited trait will undoubtedly be available in the future.

Another risk factor is the level of male hormones in the blood. It is clear that the prostate develops naturally from the stimulation of male hormones (androgens). The principal male hormone is testosterone, of which the important metabolic by-product is called dihydrotestosterone (DHT). And both these androgens are important for the development of your prostate.

Given the variability of male hormone levels, is there a relationship between hormone level and the risk of prostate cancer? Some studies suggest that there is, while others do not support this conclusion. Once again, there are no firm scientific conclusions on this association.

Several studies have looked at the differences in hormone levels, or for the genetic factors controlling these hormone levels, in different racial and ethnic groups to try to explain the differing susceptibilities to prostate cancer. A study published in the medical journal *Lancet* several years ago compared the hormone levels of Japanese men with those in both black and white American men. Remember, the incidence of prostate cancer is lower in Japa-

Table 1.
Age-Related Risk of Prostate Cancer for American Men

Current Age	Likelihood of Diagnosis This Year
40–44	1 in 58,824
45–49	1 in 13,158
50–54	1 in 2,667
55–59	1 in 874
60–64	1 in 348
65–69	1 in 174
70–74	1 in 115
75–79	1 in 90
80–84	1 in 80

Adapted from *Harvard Health Letter.* Total risk-associated factors: age, race and ethnic background, family history/genetic blueprint, dietary factors, and hormonal variations.

nese men. The most striking finding in the study was that levels of the 5-alpha reductase, the enzyme that converts testosterone to dihydrotestosterone, were lower in Japanese men than American men, either black or white. This preliminary finding suggests that the difference in incidence of prostate cancer between Japanese and American men may be partially due to relatively different levels of this enzyme among populations.

As a general rule, you are at much greater risk for prostate cancer if you have one or more male relatives who have the disease. The more close-bloodline relatives you have who have been diagnosed with the disease, the greater your risk is. Incidentally, you may want to ask your doctor about ongoing national research studies that are investigating the genetic makeup of men from families in which prostate cancer is common.

Prevention

What does all this information mean, and can you use it to lower your risk for developing prostate cancer? At present we cannot change our genes, and since our genetic blueprint plays a large role in determining whether or not we will develop prostate cancer, part of our fate is already determined. The role that diet and lifestyle play is probably important but difficult to quantify.

In terms of general health, regular exercise and a diet low in fat make a lot of sense. Diets that include tomato products may well be preventive, but it is too early to judge their true value. There is also currently a great deal of interest in phytoestrogens, naturally occurring plant chemicals, which may play a preventive role. These chemicals are most abundantly found in soy products, which form a large portion of traditional Asian diets. Their preventive value is still uncertain.

Vitamins, including beta-carotene, a vitamin A relative, and vitamin D, are still of uncertain value in prostate cancer prevention. The roles of other naturally occurring nutrients in our diets need to be studied.

Chemoprevention, a more active prevention strategy using drug intervention, is a very exciting area of research. With the knowledge that the male hormone (principally testosterone) is probably essential to the development of prostate cancer, drugs that decrease male hormone levels may be beneficial in preventing the disease. Drugs that may be valuable as chemoprevention agents include finasteride (Proscar). These drugs block the enzyme 5-alpha reductase, which converts testosterone into dihydrotestosterone, the most potent male hormone. The role finasteride will play is being researched. Unfortunately, the blocking of the 5-alpha reductase causes side effects.[1]

You should certainly investigate the exciting new field of diet and lifestyle change as a cancer-prevention strategy. We are all aware that quitting smoking, reducing alcohol consumption, cutting back on saturated fat, controlling weight, and increasing exercise are health-promoting steps. Will these measures protect you from prostate cancer? It's too early to know with any degree of scientific certainty. We do know that these healthy habits reduce the risk of heart disease. So what have you got to lose by getting on the healthy lifestyle bandwagon?

3

What Is Prostate Cancer?

Before focusing on the characteristics of prostate cancers, let's review some basics about cancer. Even though you've probably done your best to avoid thinking about cancer for most of your life, it is beneficial to be educated about the disease.

What Is Cancer?

Cancer, in its broadest sense, is characterized by two properties. One is an uncontrolled growth of cells leading to a tumor or mass of malignant cells. The other is a cancer's inherent tendency to invade other structures and to "metastasize" — to spread beyond the original site — through gaining access to blood vessels and lymph channels, and thus reach distant parts of your body.

This is the widest possible definition of cancer and includes malignant conditions as different as leukemia, melanoma, and prostate cancer. As we shall see, the rate of growth and the tendency to spread beyond the site of origin through metastasis — what we call a cancer's aggressiveness — varies greatly from one type of cancer to another. Indeed, cancer can be characterized medically in multiple ways and at multiple levels of organization, all the way from changes in the molecular structure of a single cell's deoxyribonucleic acid (DNA) genetic code to a visible tumor mass.

At the Molecular Level

Cancer can be looked at as a disease arising at the submicroscopic level of the cell's genetic code. Today we readily use terms such as DNA, genes, and genetic mutation, often forgetting that the science of molecular biology, on which modern genetic research is based, is only a few decades old. This new appreciation of the complex process of cellular genetics — found in the dense net of coded DNA molecules in the nuclei of the billions of cells that make up our bodies — has led us to a much greater understanding of cancer's nature.

We now know that cancer generally results from a succession of small changes beginning in the DNA of a single cell's nucleus. Most of the body's cells reproduce repeatedly during the lifetime through a process called mitosis. Responding to subtle chemical signals, a cell's DNA divides and replicates. The nucleus splits in two and the replicated DNA is shared between the two resulting "daughter" cells, or clones.

Cellular growth and eventual cell death (apoptosis) are an ongoing and usually balanced process. What we call specialized tissue normally follows predictable growth patterns. Your kidney cells reproduce at a standard rate as needed, and these organs do not grow beyond normal size and density unless put under some type of stress. The same is true for the other tissue systems and organs in your body. The study of molecular biology has proved that cellular replication and tissue maintenance is an extremely complex process.

However, accidents often happen during this intricate process. DNA is a complex molecule and can be damaged by a variety of agents, including the ultraviolet radiation in sunlight and by chemicals, both natural and manmade. And we know there are many unexplained factors that cause breaks, or mutations, in the cells' DNA genetic code. In fact, genetic mutation is a process as old as cellular life on this planet. Given the unique ability of the DNA molecule to self-replicate, all evolution from lower to higher species involved such DNA changes.

Mistakes causing alterations in DNA can occur during mitosis. Infrequent, random-change events may be repaired by the cell itself, but also they may accumulate with the aging process.

There are specific types of DNA mutations that we call the initiators of cancer. Our current understanding of the cancer process suggests that mutations in the genetic code at important places on the "supercoiled" DNA molecule will set the stage for the eventual uncontrolled — malignant — replication of that cell. Once the initiator events have damaged DNA in a certain way, other factors come into play — this is called the promotion phase. During promotion, further mutations may or may not occur. A cell that is primed for cancerous overgrowth will do so at some point during or after the initiating DNA-damaging events have taken place.

All cancers share this carcinogenesis process. After initiation has occurred and the promotion phase is operative, cancers vary markedly both in their growth rates and in their ability to invade surrounding structures and spread through metastasis. This is an important issue and pertains to the natural history, or variable behavior, of prostate cancer.

With the powerful techniques of molecular biology, we can recognize a cell as being cancerous by detecting certain significant gene alterations, sometimes long before the cell would have begun the typical uncontrolled growth of malignancy. However, I don't want to give you the false hope that we have the ability to take an individual cell from your body, test it for abnormal genetic activity, and warn you that the suspect tissue — your prostate or a section of your colon, for example — should be removed as a preventive step. This degree of detection sensitivity may be available in the future.

At the Cellular or Tissue Level

On a slightly larger scale, at the cellular or tissue level, pathologists can examine samples called biopsy specimens under the microscope. Pathologists look for abnormal features in these samples that are characteristic of cancer. In a microscopic examination of a biopsy specimen, the cells may appear particularly bizarre in shape and size when compared to nonmalignant tissue. The nuclei of cancerous cells where the DNA genetic material is carried may also appear particularly prominent. Cancerous cells are typically arranged in recognizably disorganized fashion, the result of uncontrolled growth.

Grading Cancer

Close scrutiny of biopsy tissue results in the pathological grading of a cancer. This is an assessment of cellular disorganization and is often described in terms of well-differentiated versus poorly differentiated cancer cells. The term differentiated implies the degree that a tissue has altered in appearance compared to what noncancerous tissue should look like. Under the microscope, normal, nonmalignant prostate cells are organized in a predictable fashion. They have clearly defined architecture, cell structure, and easily identifiable nuclei: the architectural integrity of the tissue appears to be normal.

In prostate cancer, the cellular architecture varies greatly.[1] Well-differentiated cancers are those in which the cells are similar to, but distinct from, normal tissue. Poorly differentiated cancer cells appear much more diverse in size and shape. As the level (grade) of malignancy increases, cancer cells become increasingly bizarre in appearance. It becomes more difficult to recognize the tissue of origin as the cancer becomes less differentiated.

In biopsy samples, these highly malignant cells have often lost all appearance of glandular tissue and have infiltrated widely through stromal tissue. For example, if a urologist takes a biopsy sample from your prostate and the tissue is normal, the pathologist will immediately identify the typical structure of the cells. But if a sample is taken from a high-grade malignant prostate tumor, the examining pathologist initially might have trouble identifying that the source of the tissue was the prostate. Pathologists, however, are trained to recognize these telltale patterns of malignancy in cancers affecting different organs and tissues, including prostate epithelial tissue.

Detecting cancer in a biopsy through this manner is called pathological confirmation — that is, a trained pathologist sees the unmistakable visual evidence of cancer. However, in the microscopic examination of a biopsy sample, a pathologist can identify relatively few cancerous cells among hundreds or even thousands of normal cells. This represents a different situation than a physician discovering a large, palpable, cancerous tumor that is readily seen or felt, which contains trillions of malignant cells.

With prostate cancer, there can be a wide discrepancy between what a pathologist calls a cancer and what clinicians may diagnose when studying X-rays or examining you.[2]

The Gleason Score

From a microscopic biopsy examination, a pathological grade is established on a scale called the Gleason score. This score provides a means of estimating the aggressiveness of your malignancy. The scale has five grades (sometimes called histologic or cellular appearance patterns), with Gleason score 1 being the lowest level or grade of malignancy (or aggressiveness), and 5 being the highest.

Patterns (grades) 1 and 2 describe well-differentiated cancer cells. Pattern 3 is used to describe "moderately differentiated" malignant cells. Patterns 4 and 5 categorize poorly differentiated cells. A Gleason pattern 1 cancer shows the lowest level of malignancy, with pattern 5 showing the highest.[3]

Since many tumors are a hodge-podge of patterns, the apparent grades of the two dominant patterns the pathologist sees in a sample are added together, giving rise to a final score, for example, 4 + 3 = Gleason score 7, and 3 + 5 = Gleason score 8 (*see figures 9 and 10*). Therefore, pathologists may determine the degree of aggressiveness of the prostate cancer — or other

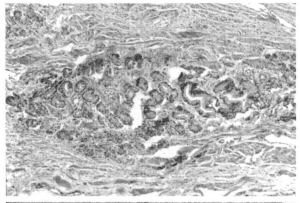

9. Biopsy sample indicating prostate cancer with mixed Gleason grades 2 and 5

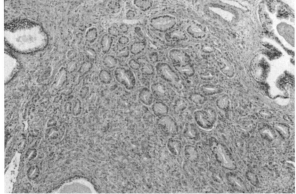

10. Biopsy sample indicating prostate cancer with mixed Gleason grades 3 through 4 and 5

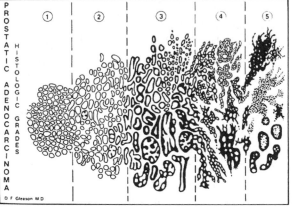

12. Histologic grades of prostatic adenocarcinoma: horizontal representation of the Gleason grading system for prostate cancer indicating typical "spill over" between grades

HISTOLOGIC GRADING OF PROSTATIC ADENOCARCINOMA

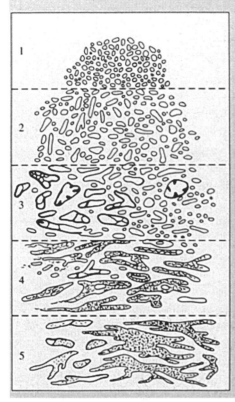

1
- sharply circumscribed aggregate of small, closely packed, uniform glands

2
- greater variation in glandular size
- more stroma between glands
- more infiltrative margins

3
- further variation in glandular size
- glands more widely dispersed in stroma
- distinctly infiltrative margins, with loss of circumscription

4
- "fused gland" pattern—irregular masses of neoplastic glands coalescing and branching
- infiltration of prostatic stroma

5
- diffusely infiltrating tumor cells with only occasional gland formation

Adapted from Gleason, 1977

11. Histologic grading of prostatic adenocarcinoma: the Gleason grading system for prostate cancer. Grade 1 (top) represents well-differentiated cancer cells; grade 5 (bottom) represents poorly differentiated cancer cells. (Courtesy, Merck Human Health Division)

malignancy — from the biopsy samples they examine (*see figures 11 and 12*).

Some physicians use grading systems other than the Gleason scale. Although these systems can be very useful, the Gleason score is the grading system used by most pathologists and clinicians.

The Stages of Prostate Cancer — The Extent of Disease

The stage of a prostate cancer relates to its size and the degree to which it has spread. The system of prostate cancer staging was developed by comparing groups of patients whose tumors share certain characteristics.

Remember that grade and stage are descriptive terms, estimates of the malignant nature and extent of a cancer. So, if you are diagnosed with prostate cancer, don't be surprised or unduly alarmed if the grade and stage estimated by one pathologist or urologist varies slightly from that of others with whom you have sought a second opinion.

Prostate cancer staging can be divided into localized (early) and metastatic (advanced) disease, with localized prostate cancer patients having no overt evidence of metastatic disease; the cancer appears to be completely confined within the prostate.

In contrast, metastatic prostate cancer patients have overt evidence of metastases, which are malignant "seeds" that have spread from the prostate to sites elsewhere in the body. Metastases often reach the lymph nodes located on your lymphatic network that contains the lymphocytes, the defending warrior cells of the immune system. Metastatic prostate cancer also spreads to the bones. Bone scans or CT (computerized tomography) scans are done to determine whether the cancer has spread (*see figure 13*).

Depending on their age, men who suffer from metastatic disease generally have a compromised life expectancy. Men with localized prostate cancer have a much better prognosis and stand a good chance of being fully cured and of living normal life spans.

Localized and metastatic prostate cancer traditionally have been grouped into one of four stages in the Whitmore-Jewett staging system. The stages range from A through D, with substages for more precise definition. Early, or localized, prostate cancer is divided into stages A, B, and C.

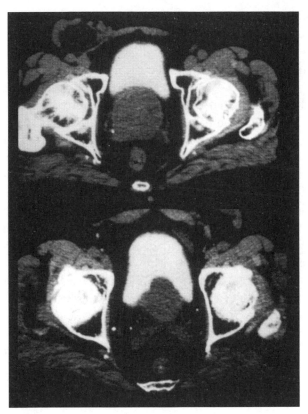

13. CT scans of nonmalignant prostate with BPH and healthy seminal vesicles; lower view is at higher magnification (Courtesy, Merck Human Health Division)

Stage A is diagnosed in connection with a TURP (transurethral resection of the prostate), usually performed to alleviate serious symptoms of BPH. In these cases, prostate cancer is not anticipated and is discovered incidentally by a pathologist examining the tissue removed from the transition zone during the BPH surgery. Because more urologists are controlling BPH with prescription drugs rather than surgery, this form of prostate cancer diagnosis is now less common. But if a TURP-related pathological diagnosis is made, the cancer is often stage A, arising in the transition zone. Cancers discovered this way, particularly those that are low grade (well-differentiated cells) and low volume (only a small amount of tissue examined containing cancer) — so-called A1 prostate cancer — are sometimes referred to as incidental because they are detected only in connection with TURP surgery.

The more common route to prostate cancer diagnosis today is an abnormal PSA and/or DRE. After the detection of an elevated PSA level, a man undergoes a biopsy, from which a pathologist can detect and grade a cancer.

Staging systems are frequently used by physicians to classify the extent of cancer and to communicate with their colleagues on what the gland feels like in order to determine the prognosis and the appropriate therapy.

Stage B prostate cancers are those that the physician can detect by touch (palpate) during a DRE. The doctor feels a characteristic hard nodule or gritty consistency in one side or lobe of the gland — in the peripheral zone — beneath the thin, smooth capsule of the prostate. This harder tissue can vary in size, from the diameter of a grape seed to a larger mass involving the entire gland.

We further divide the stage of localized prostate cancer by degree of involvement of the gland. Stage B1 is generally palpable in one half of one of the posterior lobes of the prostate. Stage B2 are cancers that appear to be present throughout most of one posterior lobe. Stage B3 cancer is present in both posterior lobes. Stage C is characterized by tumors that, when felt during a DRE, appear to extend beyond the confines of the prostate into other structures, either into the seminal vesicles, which are the pouches that collect the semen after the prostate produces it, or into surrounding tissues.

Men with overt evidence of metastatic disease have stage D prostate cancer. The metastatic spread of disease to lymph nodes within the pelvis is called stage D1. Stage D2 is the spread beyond the lymph nodes to bone, the most common site of metastatic disease in prostate cancer.

Stage D1 prostate cancer in general has a much more favorable outlook than stage D2 disease. In stage D1, the survival is frequently greater than five years. But in stage D2, survival generally is only a few years after diagnosis.

Most patients diagnosed with prostate cancer today, however, are categorized by a newer method called the Tumor Nodes Metastasis (TNM) staging system, which physicians prefer to the Whitmore-Jewett because of its greater precision.

The TNM stage T1 cancer corresponds to the Whitmore-Jewett stage A cancer but includes the subcategory T1c. This comprises a growing number of men who are symptom free and first manifest their cancer in the form of an elevated PSA level. So a man with stage T1c disease often has a normal prostate by DRE examination, but has an elevated PSA, which leads to the biopsy that reveals pathological evidence of prostate cancer. You may fit this pattern. (You may also hear a physician describe a stage T1c cancer as a B0 tumor, a subcategory of the Whitmore-Jewett system.)

Stage T2 prostate cancers are like those of stage B: this stage is palpable to the doctor during the DRE exam, and the cancerous cells are found in either one or both lobes of the prostate.

Stage T3 prostate cancers are parallel to stage C cancers, and so forth; they are palpable beyond the confines of the prostate, often in the seminal vesicles. (See table 2 for comparison of the TNM and Whitmore-Jewett staging systems.)

I urge you to keep in mind that the staging of prostate cancer is not very accurate, unless the prostate and the nearby lymph nodes are removed during radical prostatectomy surgery. Staging that occurs after the prostate is removed, the pathological stage, is distinct from clinical staging. Surgical removal of the prostate permits more precise staging than DRE or imaging with ultrasound, CT scan, or magnetic resonance imaging (MRI). This pathological examination permits exact staging into stages A, B, or C (or T1, T2, and T3) because the pathologist can dissect the entire prostate and surrounding tissue. Similar to clinical staging, which helps determine prognosis and type of therapy, postsurgical staging helps to accurately determine whether the cancer is confined to the prostate and surrounding structures.

However, short of surgically removing the gland, we must depend on less accurate staging examinations, including the DRE, ultrasound imaging, CT scan, or MRI, all of which are subject to divergent interpretation. With the DRE, for example, the physician must define the extent of the tumor by touch alone.

If you have been diagnosed with Whitmore-Jewett stages A or B prostate cancer (TNM stages T1 and T2), you probably have an excellent prognosis. With treatment — usually radical prostatectomy or radiation therapy — your cancer at this stage has a high likelihood of being cured. The prognosis of A and B cancers is influenced by other factors that are known (for example, grade, PSA level) and perhaps by additional yet unknown factors.

If you receive a diagnosis of stage C cancer (TNM stage T3), which by definition extends beyond the prostate, your chance of completely ridding your body of this malignancy is relatively low. And prostate cancer at this stage is often associated with recurrence following treatment. But you should not give in to despair after diagnosis because, as I will discuss in detail, you can live for many years with stage C prostate cancer.

Determining the pathological grade and clinical stage of prostate cancer is a critical step in establishing the best course of noncurative treatment. The physicians who made your diagnosis most certainly did their best possible job, but if you have any doubt, get a second opinion. If you belong to a health maintenance organization (HMO), this might involve burdensome paperwork. Also, some health insurance companies might balk at paying for a review of the biopsy or a review of your status by other physicians. But most health care programs do provide for second opinions. And, when it comes to a diagnosis of prostate cancer, you should stand up for your right to a second and even a third opinion before deciding on treatment.

Table 2. The Stages of Prostate Cancer

TNM	Whitmore-Jewett	Description
T1	A	Cancer unpalpable in DRE
T1a	A1	Less than 5 percent of sample malignant and low-grade
T1b	A2	More than 5 percent of sample malignant and/or not low-grade
T1c	(B0)	PSA elevated, not palpable
T2	B	Tumor digitally palpable in DRE; organ confined
T2a	B1	Confined to one lobe of gland < 1.5 cm
T2b	B2	Confined to one lobe of gland > 1.5 cm
T2c		Palpable in both lobes
T3	C	Locally extensive cancer
	C1	Penetration of prostate capsule
	C2	Seminal vesicle involvement
T4	C3	Tumor extension to adjacent organs
Tx, N1, or M1	D	Distant metastases
Tx, N1, M0	D1	Pelvic lymph node involvement
Tx, Nx, M1	D2	Metastasis to distant sites other than lymph nodes (bone)

Case History: Bill J.

Last year, a couple named Bill and Susan J. came to my office at the Dana-Farber Cancer Institute in Boston for a consultation.

Bill had just turned 55. But like many health-conscious professionals of his generation, he looked years younger. His wife, Susan, an energetic woman of 50, sat anxiously beside Bill as we discussed his situation.

Bill is an executive of a computer firm in the high-tech region west of Boston. During a routine medical exam three weeks earlier, his doctor found him in seemingly excellent overall health. His serum cholesterol was under 200 and his blood pressure was normal. He showed no evidence of cardiovascular disease. As a nonsmoker who took only an occasional social drink and watched his diet, while mitigating the stress of his job with regular exercise and relaxing hobbies, Bill was the ideal middle-aged patient.

His doctor had drawn the PSA test. When the laboratory results indicated that Bill had an elevated PSA level for a man his age — 4.3 nanograms per milliliter (ng/ml) of blood — his physician was concerned. Bill returned for a reexamination, which entailed another digital rectal examination and a repeat PSA.

Bill's prostate had the normal enlargement for a man in his sixth decade of life, and the gland appeared healthy due to its smooth texture. But because the PSA level was still elevated, the doctor recommended that Bill see a urologist, who confirmed the findings of Bill's doctor and ordered a transrectal ultrasound exam and a prostate biopsy.

The biopsy is a procedure involving a rectal ultrasound probe that images the prostate while the physician guides a hollow needle into the prostate to extract small tissue core samples from different regions of the gland. These samples are then examined by a pathologist.

Four days after the biopsy, Bill drove back to the urologist, terrified of learning the results. His fear was justified: one of the biopsy samples showed microscopic evidence of prostate cancer in the upper portion of the right side of the gland, Gleason grade $2 + 3 = 5$.

At that time, Bill requested a consultation with me to discuss his best treatment options. I was glad that his wife joined him, as the decisions he needed to make would affect them both for the rest of their lives. Prostate cancer, like other cancers, is a disease that affects a family, not only an individual. The Joneses were seeking reassurance at the most frightening time of their married life. Just a few weeks earlier they had assumed Bill was healthy, and yet now he had cancer, harsh news for any patient and his family.

How, Bill asked, could this cancer have suddenly appeared when he had no symptoms and no family history of the disease? Did something in the environment or in his diet cause it? What were his treatment options? Would the surgical and radiation procedures they had heard of lead to the unwelcome side effects of permanent sexual impotence and urinary incontinence?

Because Bill was diagnosed with cancer, both he and Susan had to confront these issues. Though Bill was used to making difficult business decisions, he clearly was not prepared to face this most difficult decision of his personal life. Bill's urologist had given him a pamphlet that briefly described the standard treatment options: radical prostatectomy, radiation therapy, and the monitoring process called watchful waiting, or observation.

In discussing these options with his wife, Bill, like many men, was preoccupied with the negative side effects of both surgery and radiation therapy. Susan was also distraught. They had been married for almost twenty-five years and shared a close physical relationship. Like most men, Bill was reluctant to discuss impotence as a side effect of treatment, but I knew the issue haunted him. Susan frankly admitted that the prospect of her otherwise healthy and vigorous husband becoming permanently impotent, as well as possibly incontinent of urine, was horrible.

Bill focused his anxiety on urinary incontinence. He and Susan were avid golfers. They were planning their retirement in the Southwest around golf and their other shared hobbies — whitewater rafting and skiing. Bill needed to know if the side effects of treatment — especially urinary incontinence — would make these activities impossible. After he'd raised these concerns, Bill found the words that epitomized his greatest fear: "Is this prostate cancer going to kill me?"

I had explanations for Bill and Susan's questions and information that would allay their fear and confusion. First I assured them, "You don't have to rush the decision on what treatment is best for you. This tumor isn't going to become life-threatening tomorrow."

They were relieved to know they had time to weigh treatment options. I carefully explained the different types of treatments that are most appropriate for localized prostate cancer (cancer that is still confined within the gland). These treatments include radical prostatectomy surgery; external beam radiation therapy; radiation therapy using implants placed directly into the tumor; and cryosurgery, which involves freezing the cancerous prostate cells. Each of these treatments has its benefits, risks, and side effects. The one factor they have in common is that they are considered curative: they each have the potential of killing or ridding the body of all the cancer cells before the disease has spread beyond the prostate gland.

Bill and Susan decided to proceed with radiation implants: they believed that, despite the relatively limited experience with this type of treatment, it offered Bill the best balance of risk and benefit. Specifically, radiation implants (discussed in Chapter 8) may pose less risk of impotence or urinary incontinence than surgery yet may be curative.

4

The Natural History
of Prostate Cancer

Cancer's Natural History

Cancer results from a succession of minor changes in the cell's genetic material. When these changes accumulate, cells increasingly acquire the characteristics of cancer: abnormal shape and size and varying degrees of uncontrolled growth. The cells may eventually become a tumor, with a grade, a volume, and the likelihood of spreading, or metastasizing, to other parts of the body. In different malignant tumors, the speed of this genetic change can vary greatly. This is part of what we call a particular cancer's natural history. It is vital that you understand this concept in order to best plan your treatment strategy with your doctor.

Prostate cancer behaves differently than other cancers, and each tumor in every individual behaves differently — thus the natural history is variable. Unfortunately, the natural history of prostate cancer is more difficult to predict than that of other diseases. For example, a typically aggressive malignant lung tumor poses a threat of rapid, deadly metastatic spread, and therefore a diagnosis of localized lung cancer generally calls for immediate medical treatment, usually involving surgery. Prostate cancer's speed of progression, although generally slower than other types of cancer, is simply not as predictable.

Prostate Cancer's Natural History

Prostate cancer shares some features with other cancers but differs in several significant ways. Most importantly, there is a greater disparity between clinical prostate cancer and what we call pathological prostate cancer. Pathological prostate cancer is what a pathologist sees in the microscopic examination of a biopsy. Clinical prostate cancer is what the clinician sees upon examining you.

A small cancerous tumor can exist in the prostate for years without presenting any symptoms, and it may *never* be detected or pose a problem. Your physician may feel no evidence of a tumor when examining your prostate during the digital rectal examination. However, when a pathologist examines a biopsy of this cancerous tissue under the microscope, the cells will show obvious cancerous characteristics.

This was the case for Bill J. His DRE suggested a healthy prostate with a normal degree of enlargement for a man Bill's age. But after the biopsy, the pathologist had more than an adequate sample of cancerous tissue to confirm his diagnosis. Bill's Gleason score of 5, however, suggested a tumor of intermediate aggressiveness. With the use of the PSA blood test, followed by biopsy, this pattern of cancer is found more frequently.

Some of the cancers detected may lead to problems if left untreated. On the other hand, some cancers detected may not be clinically important — that is, they may never cause a problem.

A dramatic discrepancy between pathological prostate cancer and clinical prostate cancer has been found by pathologists who perform autopsies and examine the prostates of men who have died of causes other than prostate cancer: they often find evidence of cancerous cells in the prostate. This "autopsy cancer" is seen in about 30 percent of men over the age of 50 who undergo postmortem examination. And this percentage certainly increases with age. Considering this, a staggering statistic emerges: more than 8 million men in the United States probably have prostate cancer. And as the baby boom generation reaches middle age, that number will only increase. Such evidence underlies the medical axiom "More men die *with* prostate cancer than *from* it."

Of the prostate cancers that pathologists detect in postmortem examinations, only a small fraction appear to have had the potential for aggressive growth. This is a critical point. So-called "latent" prostate cancers often exist in the gland for many years before they are detected or cause problems. And the biggest controversy in the treatment of prostate cancer is deciding which cancers are clinically important.

Probably the earliest pathological manifestation of prostate cancer is a transformation of the epithelial cells called prostatic intra-epithelial neoplasia, or PIN. This condition produces cells that a pathologist can recognize microscopically and which many clinicians believe is the precursor to prostate cancer. But the condition is not cancer because PIN cells have not yet invaded the stromal tissue or the prostate's external capsule. And, to the best of medical knowledge, PIN does not have the potential to metastasize. PIN cells presumably have undergone some but not all the genetic changes needed to become prostate cancer. PIN may co-exist in the same gland with prostate cancer. Alternatively, it may predate prostate cancer by years. It is also possible that a person with PIN may never develop prostate cancer.

Pathologists familiar with PIN will grade this abnormality from low- to high-grade. Given the increased number of biopsies following PSA screening, more PIN is being detected. But we do not yet know the importance of PIN. It is not full-blown cancer and does not require treatment. The existence of PIN should not change the physician's management of a man's prostate cancer in any way. In my opinion, men who have undergone a biopsy in which PIN — but no carcinoma — has been detected should probably join the group of patients who have consulted with their physicians and opted for watchful waiting. This involves annual PSA tests and DREs. But if you have PIN and have also been diagnosed with prostate cancer, you need not be alarmed that the PIN will somehow make your cancer more dangerous.

Almost all of what we normally call prostate cancer — prostate carcinoma — is a malignancy that arises from the epithelial or glandular component of the prostate. There are some other rare types of cancers, however — sarcomas and small-cell carcinomas — that may originate in the prostate from nonglandular tissue. But the vast majority of prostate cancer are common adenocarcinomas (*adeno* meaning glandlike).

Typical prostate cancer is recognized by malignant epithelial cells invading stromal tissue. This may occur in either side of the gland in discrete areas. If large enough, the malignancy can form a nodule. Or the invasion of stromal tissue by malignant epithelial cells may be diffuse throughout your prostate, in which case the cancer may not be palpable or detectable during a DRE. When invasion of cancerous cells into the stromal tissue occurs, the possibility for metastasis exists.

We do not know how long the conversion from a normal prostate epithelium to a malignant epithelium takes, or the time frame in which invasion of the surrounding stromal tissue occurs. Our best estimates are that this process occurs very slowly, over many years.

As with other carcinomas, prostate cancer results from an accumulation of genetic changes to epithelial cells. But prostate cancer may be one of the most heterogeneous of all cancers. That is, the behavior — natural history — of prostate cancer in different individuals can vary greatly. There are clearly some prostate cancers that are very aggressive and some that are quite indolent. But, at present, we don't understand all the factors that determine these characteristics.

In a simplified view of cancer in general, the growth rates of a malignant tumor begin slowly, and as genetic changes accumulate, the pace of growth increases and parallels the ability of the cells to divide uncontrollably and ultimately metastasize. This is called a tumor's metastatic potential.

By this model, a particular prostate cancer early in its natural history grows very slowly and doubles in volume only after several years. But, as it continues to grow and accumulate genetic change, the growth rate increases. This would suggest that larger cancers are growing faster than smaller ones. This association is hard to prove, however, and it may well be an inappropriate oversimplification to apply this size/growth model to every prostate cancer.

Some small prostate cancers may grow quickly and aggressively, while larger prostate cancers may remain indolent. A single prostate tumor often contains different grades of cancer. It is currently hard to predict which cancers are going to be "clinically important" and which are not. But just such an accurate prediction is probably your most important tool in deciding on a particular treatment option.

5

Screening for Prostate Cancer

Traditional Means of Detection

In the past, prostate cancer was typically discovered by a physician examining your prostate gland during a digital rectal exam and detecting a suspicious hard area, which would prompt a biopsy of the prostate. Alternatively, the disease was detected after it had spread beyond the gland to the bones and caused pain.

Your doctor would also be alerted to the possibility of prostate cancer if you complained of trouble urinating. This might indicate that a prostate cancer was growing within the gland.

Since the DRE is still an important diagnostic technique, which most of you will experience during regular physical exams, we should detail how this examination is conducted and what your physician does — and does not — learn from it. During a DRE of the prostate, your doctor will either ask you to stand and bend forward, or to lie down on your side. By inserting a gloved, lubricated finger into your rectum, he examines the posterior portion of the prostate, which is adjacent to the rectum. This isn't a comfortable procedure, but it's not unduly painful, either. Used as the sole diagnostic tool for prostate cancer, however, it isn't efficient.

Doctors have differing levels of expertise in performing the DRE. The general practitioners and internists in practice or at a typical HMO should be proficient at the examination, since they often conduct routine physical exams. Urologists have the most experience performing this exam. The physician performing your DRE should be able to distinguish a normal from an abnormal gland by size and texture. How doctors interpret the signs they detect during the examination varies. What one physician feels to be a smooth, normal gland, another might find suspiciously hard. Frankly, many physicians are not well trained in conducting the DRE.

Your doctor cannot see your prostate during a DRE, and furthermore, he or she can examine only the posterior section of the gland. Although most cancers originate in the posterior lobes, some cancers are small, diffuse, or centrally located, resulting in no palpable abnormalities. It is therefore wrong to assume that your doctor will find all prostate cancers by feeling your gland during a DRE.

Another drawback of the DRE when used alone is that by the time a prostate cancer is detectable by examination, it has often spread beyond the confines of the gland. Once this has happened, the disease usually cannot be cured.

Physicians recognize that the DRE is not a foolproof test for detecting early, curable prostate cancer.

The Prostate-Specific Antigen Test

The prostate-specific antigen (PSA) blood test arrived on the scene in 1987. The PSA was initially developed by scientists who discovered that one of the most abundant chemical components of semen was a protein we now call PSA. The PSA protein's function is as a protease or an enzyme, and it breaks down certain types of other proteins. Researchers determined that the PSA protein was present in the blood as well, and then they discovered that the PSA is exclusively produced by the epithelial (glandular) part of the prostate. No other human tissue produces this protein, hence the term "specific" in PSA.

Much of the PSA produced by the gland's cells empties into the hundreds of tiny tubes in the prostate, where it mixes with the ejaculate. A small portion is absorbed into the bloodstream; this is why it may be measured by a blood test.

A man who has not had his prostate removed produces a certain amount of PSA, which is detected in the blood. The level of PSA in the blood is normally quite low — a few *billionths* of a gram (nanograms) per milliliter (ng/ml) of blood. The level of PSA detected in the blood is usually determined by the amount of prostate glandular tissue in the body. Women do not have a prostate; they do not make PSA.

Because the prostate naturally increases in size through the benign (noncancerous) process called prostatic hyperplasia (BPH), the prostate accumulates more cells, both glandular and stromal. PSA levels generally increase with age as the prostate grows larger. Remember, BPH occurs in a significant percentage of aging men without prostate cancer, and you're probably no exception.

BPH is *common* and may elevate the PSA, and most men with elevated PSA levels do not have prostate cancer. The majority of men with high PSA levels have BPH as the cause of their above-"normal" test results (*see figure 14*).

In general, your PSA level is partially age dependent. Normal levels were established through clinical research soon after the test was developed, and though more accurate adjustments for age are being investigated, your physician most likely follows the original guidelines.

Prostatitis is another noncancerous cause of elevated PSA (other than BPH). Prostatitis causes inflammation that can raise the PSA level dramatically because inflamed glandular tissue allows more of the protein to gain access to the blood. A 45-year-old man without BPH might have an extremely elevated PSA level (over 50.0 ng/ml) if he is suffering a bout of acute prostatitis. Chronic prostatitis, or a condition wherein someone has multiple bouts of prostatitis, might cause sustained mild PSA elevations. You should be knowledgeable about prostatitis — either acute or chronic — if you have it. If you've had prostatitis, defi-

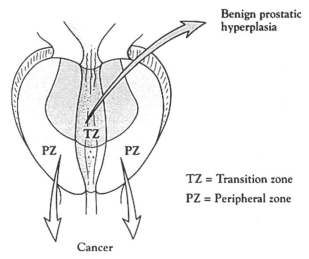

Benign prostatic
hyperplasia

TZ = Transition zone
PZ = Peripheral zone

Cancer

14. Zones of the prostate with typical locations of BPH
and prostate cancer (Courtesy, Merck Human Health Division)

nitely tell your physician about it before undergoing PSA screening for prostate cancer.

Although BPH or chronic prostatitis often cause mild elevations in the PSA, prostate cancer — not these benign conditions — is most frequently the cause of a sustained and markedly elevated PSA level (greater than 10.00 ng/ml). The only reliable way to distinguish prostate cancer from noncancerous causes of an elevated PSA is by biopsy.

Remember that your PSA level correlates with the number of glandular prostate cells present in your body. And since prostate cancer is a malignancy of these glandular cells, which proliferate through the type of uncontrolled growth we discussed earlier, the level of PSA in a man with prostate cancer correlates with the total number of malignant prostate epithelial cells (what doctors call the volume of the tumor).

If the malignant prostate tumor is large — occupying an entire lobe or even both lobes — it is very possible that the cancer has undergone metastasis. So if you have prostate cancer, your level of PSA provides important information about the likelihood that the cancer has spread, especially if that level is greatly elevated. Moreover, malignant prostate epithelial cells that have spread through metastasis to sites beyond the gland continue to produce PSA even after the prostate has been surgically removed or destroyed through radiation therapy, cryosurgery, or microwaves.

The chances that you have the disease will increase in proportion to your PSA level. If you have mildly elevated PSA, you are far less likely to have prostate cancer than someone with a very elevated level. For example, a 65-year-old man with a PSA of 4.5 ng/ml might simply have BPH. But a man with a PSA of 10.0 ng/ml almost certainly has prostate cancer, in the absence of prostatitis.

Age-Adjusted PSA

Because your PSA level increases as you age and as the size of your prostate increases, the significance of a slightly elevated PSA level in a 45-year-old is quite different than a similar level in a 75-year-old man (*see table 3*). Thus, a PSA of 4.2 in a 45-year old is very suspicious — barring evidence of unusually extensive BPH or of prostatitis. In a man who is 75, such a level is likely to be normal.

There is increasing evidence that the range of a healthy man's PSA levels should be much different for younger men than for older men. Your PSA level must be looked at in the context of your age and the size of your prostate gland. If you are under 50, a PSA value higher than 2.5 ng/ml might be reason for concern. In your fifties, a PSA value of above 3.5 ng/ml might be of concern; 5.5 ng/ml when you reach your sixties; and 6.5 ng/ml when you are over 70.

Since your PSA level can vary greatly with your prostate size and degree of BPH (if any), which are often dependent on age, you should ask your physician after PSA screening: "Is this PSA level appropriate for the size of my prostate and my age?"

The perception of the PSA as the infallible blood test for prostate cancer is misleading.

The PSA test measures the amount of a protein in the blood detected by a laboratory process called radio-immuno assay. A variety of tumor markers from other types of cancer also utilize this technology. Currently laboratories use several immuno-assay techniques that employ different antibodies to identify the PSA protein.

Because of these different techniques, there may be slight variability in the PSA level number among different labs. This may be quite confusing to you as a patient or to your doctor. In an effort to maintain consistency, your physician should try to use a particular laboratory so that the results follow a predictable pattern.

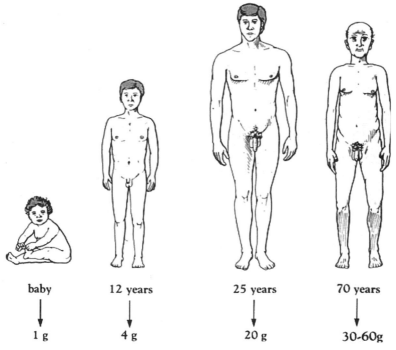

baby	12 years	25 years	70 years
↓	↓	↓	↓
1 g	4 g	20 g	30-60g

15. Prostate gland weight versus age (Courtesy, Merck Human Health Division)

Table 3. Age-Adjusted PSA Values

Determining normal PSA values can be difficult and confusing given the common condition of benign enlargement of the prostate in men over 45. The *upper* levels of age-adjusted PSA values are listed below. Age-adjusted PSA values *above* these levels should be reason for further evaluation.

Age	PSA Value	Comment
40–49	1.0–2.4 ng/ml*	Normal upper limit depends on degree of individual BPH
50–59	3.4 ng/ml*	Age-normal BPH should be verified by DRE
60–69	5.4 ng/ml*	Age-normal BPH should be verified
70–79	6.4 ng/ml*	Age-normal BPH should be verified

*In the absence of prostatitis

This can help prevent undue anxiety brought on by false high readings, and also prevent unnecessary medical procedures triggered by such readings. Don't hesitate to ask your doctor if he or she is satisfied with the consistency of the lab's PSA results.

Researchers have also recently discovered that a man's PSA level can be elevated if he has ejaculated within the two days prior to having blood drawn for the test. Dr. Joseph E. Oesterling, director of the University of Michigan's Prostate Institute, studied PSA levels from the blood tests of sixty-four men who ranged in age from 49 to 79. Oesterling's researchers measured blood PSA levels in the men over several days, during which they all ejaculated. The PSA levels of fifty-six of these men increased significantly and remained elevated for at least six hours after ejaculation. This increase averaged 0.8 ng/ml, enough to elevate the PSA levels of 15 percent of the men over the 4.0 ng/ml normal level. The PSA levels returned to the individuals' true normal level forty-eight hours after ejaculation.

Therefore, if you know you're going to have blood drawn for a PSA level, it is best to refrain from ejaculation for forty-eight hours before the test. If you have ejaculated within two days, mention this to your doctor. If you already have been tested within forty-eight hours of ejaculation and your level was elevated by 0.8 or less, discuss this with your doctor.

New PSA Tests

Certain antibodies can discriminate between two types of PSA in the blood. One type of PSA is attached, or "bound," to another serum protein, alpha 1 antichymotrypsin. The other type of PSA circulates freely from that protein. Research suggests that the determination of what proportion of PSA is bound and what proportion is free helps to distinguish PSA elevations caused by BPH from PSA elevations caused by prostate cancer. This is because the PSA that is bound to the other blood protein might be more prevalent in men with prostate cancer than in men who simply have elevated PSA due to BPH. If your physician reports that you have an elevated PSA, ask whether it would be useful to determine the ratio between the bound and free components of the PSA with this new assay. I have found this test to be particularly helpful if the proportion of free PSA is very low (less than 10 percent), which suggests the presence of prostate cancer.

Another new PSA test is the reverse-transcriptase polymerase chain reaction (RT-PCR) test. This is not simply a measure of the PSA protein in the blood, but is meant to detect tumor cells in the blood. While not a screening test, the RT-PCR might be useful if you have already been diagnosed with prostate cancer. I return to the RT-PCR for PSA test in Chapter 6.

The PSA and Prostate Cancer Diagnosis — Screening

In the past few years we have learned that PSA testing will definitely improve the detection of prostate cancer.[1]

We know that physicians using the PSA can detect prostate cancers that would otherwise be undetected through the DRE alone. This is because the PSA will help find cancers that cannot be felt during the DRE.

Research also shows that, if physicians use both the PSA and the DRE together, the ability to detect a cancer is about three times greater than if the DRE is used alone. At present, the optimal means to detect prostate cancer is by combining the PSA and DRE.

In addition to detecting diffuse cancers (cancers that don't grow as a mass, but rather a streaming fashion through the gland) that are not palpable by a DRE, use of the PSA test may find cancerous tumors too small to be palpable. The PSA, particularly when used with the DRE, is a very sensitive test.

Today, in the average population of men over 50 who undergo prostate cancer screening, about 20 percent will have some abnormality, either an abnormal PSA or DRE, and between 2 and 6 percent will be found to have prostate cancer when biopsies are performed. So if you've been dreading taking the PSA test, be assured that you have a better than 90 percent chance of being found free of prostate cancer. These odds become less favorable as you age, of course (see table 1). Furthermore, the majority of men with a minimally elevated PSA level (in the range of 4.0 to 10.0 ng/ml) do *not* have prostate cancer. Current estimates are that only 20 percent of these men have prostate cancer. If your PSA level is over 10.0 ng/ml, however, your likelihood of having prostate cancer is greater than 50 percent.

The clinical characteristics of men found to have prostate cancer discovered only by a PSA elevation are of some interest. As noted, we were concerned that many of these cancers would be latent (undetected at the time of death), which are clinically insignificant. Although the clinical behavior of the cancers cannot be reliably predicted, most men detected with prostate cancer after their first PSA tests actually had cancers of significant volume that were not low-grade.

Because the PSA used with the DRE is a more sensitive test than the DRE used alone and can detect very small tumors that are still localized in the gland, the implication is that the screening or early detection with PSA and DRE finds cancers while they are still curable. And although there is no firm evidence that this is the case, research data is accumulating that, when the PSA and DRE are used together, the physician is more likely to detect cancers that are confined to the prostate — within the capsule of the gland — than by the DRE alone.

It is mainly on the basis of this data that two influential professional groups, the American Urological Association (a society of urologists, the physicians who most often treat prostate cancer surgically) and the American Cancer Society, have made strong recommendations for early detection. Their recommendations are to screen for prostate cancer by performing an annual DRE and PSA test in every man age 50 and above. They further recommend that African-American men and any man with a family history of prostate cancer begin this screening at the age of 40.[2]

The basis for these recommendations is rooted in the high level of suffering (morbidity) and mortality from this cancer and in two observations: screening with PSA and DRE detects more cancers and detects them earlier in their course. These recommendations also stem from the hope that screening for prostate cancer will decrease the death rate of this disease.

To you and your family, a diagnostic test that can detect organ-confined prostate cancer, the stage of the disease that is more likely curable, is an extremely valuable innovation.

Concerns about Screening

The crux of the controversy over PSA screening is that the existence of a test that detects more cancers in general — and even offers early detection of organ-confined cancers — does not necessarily translate into curing more men of their prostate cancers.[3]

Perhaps an even more important issue is that early detection leads to the diagnosis of many insignificant prostate cancers. In this sequence, you would be cured of a disease that perhaps was not actually life threatening. By this I mean that a proportion of such cancers might never have posed a significant risk to either length or quality of life.

Medicine today simply does not know if it is necessary to search for and treat all the prostate cancers that are being discovered through the current aggressive screening campaign. This may come as a surprise if you've drawn comfort from the assumption that American medicine is so advanced that most major health issues are well understood. Prostate cancer is a complicated disease. The lack of full understanding of the natural history of prostate cancer is a central factor to the overall controversy of screening.

I have not raised this question to confuse you, but rather to make you aware that you should consider all these points before you engage in the screening process.

Many prostate cancers will not cause clinical problems for years, and there are competing causes of death (heart disease, stroke), especially in elderly men. Not all prostate cancer affects longevity: the cancer may grow slowly and not spread or, in older men, may not become clinically important before they die of other causes.

We need a major national research effort similar to that undertaken for breast cancer in the 1970s and 1980s. One wide-scale research study examining the value of prostate cancer screening currently being proposed is the PLCO (prostate, lung, colon, and ovarian cancers) trial, a multiyear, nationwide project organized by the National Cancer Institute. The men in the prostate cancer trials will be screened annually for four consecutive years and then followed for an additional twelve years. Unfortunately, the results of the PLCO research will not benefit this generation of potential patients.

Although evidence for the benefits of early detection of prostate cancer are suggested but not proven, concern has been raised about screening, particularly the type of routine screening that is available today. Even before the recommendations by the American Cancer Society and the American Urologic Association were announced, the Preventive Services Task Force, an American advisory body, concluded that tests such as the PSA "are not recommended for routine screening."[4]

Those opposed to routine PSA testing are concerned because prostate cancer often has a long natural history and many men live for decades with the disease before they experience clinical problems. Therefore, the likely benefit of screening — reduced mortality — would be neutralized by other causes of death, such as heart attacks and strokes.[5]

Who Should Be Screened?

The Food and Drug Administration (FDA) did not approve the PSA assay as a prostate cancer screening test until August 1994, almost ten years after it was introduced as a monitoring test to chart the progress of the disease. However, even after the FDA approved the PSA assay as a diagnostic test, the agency refused to recommend its use for widespread screening.[6]

FDA commissioner Dr. David A. Kessler told the media, "We're approving the test because it works. But whether or not to be tested needs to be a decision between patients and their physicians."

Dr. Kessler's ambivalence about the use of the PSA as a mass prostate cancer screening tool was obvious. "You're going to be picking up more pathology," he said. "And you're going to be treating more patients. But in the end, are you going to be saving more lives?"

It is my belief that the current screening strategy involving widespread PSA assays with conjoint DRE and ultrasonically guided biopsy will decrease deaths from prostate cancer. The questions are: How dramatic a decrease will it be? Who is most likely to benefit? How can we avoid treating people who do not need to be treated?

Prostate cancer will undoubtedly require an increasing proportion of health care resources as our population ages. The average age of death from this disease is 77. But compared to death rates from heart disease, stroke, and other forms of cancer, prostate cancer kills a very small proportion of American men — on the order of 1 percent of deaths in men over 50.

In some cases, screening may save lives: this is a good reason why the combined PSA and DRE should be made available. You should understand, however, that screening may not impact your risk of dying from prostate cancer; that is, the cancer detected might not pose a risk of mortality.

If we were better able to definitively select those patients who need to be treated from those who do not, such difficult decisions would not be necessary. Presently, though, despite intensive research, we have trouble distinguishing men diagnosed with prostate cancer who must undergo treatment to save their lives from those who do not have to undergo treatment.

These principles about the nature of prostate cancer may help you and your family decide whether you should be screened.

- Prostate cancer screening may save your life.
- Prostate cancer behaves differently than other cancers. It has a unique and often unpredictable natural history.
- There is a huge pool of undetected, or latent, cancers in middle-aged and elderly men. Many men over 50 who are screened are diagnosed with prostate cancer that otherwise would not have been detected for years, if ever.
- If you undergo prostate cancer screening, you should be emotionally prepared to hear that you have prostate cancer. Medical professionals who offer routine screenings should adequately prepare you for possible diagnosis and treatment.
- Research studies on localized prostate cancer reveal that survival at five years after diagnosis is excellent, whether or not you are treated.
- When considering screening, your age is an important factor. Ask your doctor to help you estimate your life expectancy based on your current age, family medical history, and overall health.
- If you have less than ten years' life expectancy, it doesn't make sense to try to detect and treat a disease that is not likely to impact on your survival.
- If you are diagnosed with localized prostate cancer in your

late 70s or in your 80s, there is a good chance you will die with, rather than from, the disease.

- After diagnosis, you *do* have time to sort out treatment options in a calm, rational manner, without undue haste.
- Treatment is an effort to prevent the suffering of metastatic prostate cancer, which can be devastating.
- Look at screening and treatment in terms of tradeoffs — years of life saved in exchange for the consequences of treatment.

Informed Consent: A Prerequisite

Hundreds of thousands of men have PSA tests drawn without their knowledge. You may be one of them. Your physician might feel that early detection of prostate cancer is a high priority for you, or perhaps routine PSA testing is part of your HMO's general policy. But in keeping with my philosophy that patients should be informed and consent to any screening, you should have the choice of whether you want your PSA tested. You should not be screened without your knowledge or unless you've been informed about the ramifications of that test, particularly treatment options and their side effects.

Men who have a short life expectancy should *not* be screened for prostate cancer. Other men — particularly those in middle age — need to have as much information as possible so that they can make an informed decision with their doctor about whether screening and eventual treatment are appropriate for them.

Case History: Joe L.

A consultation I had last summer with Joe L. describes how I employ informed consent on a practical level.

Joe, a retired railroad worker, had just turned 70 when he asked me if he should be screened for prostate cancer. He had smoked for years and had serious cardiovascular problems and emphysema. I estimated that his life expectancy was less than ten years. I told Joe that prostate cancer was a serious health problem, and that over 40,000 men would die from it each year. He had heard these figures.

Joe's wife and daughter recommended that he be screened after they learned about General Norman Schwarzkopf's operation. I explained that the PSA assay is *not* a sure-fire blood test for prostate cancer. If Joe's PSA was high, his doctor would probably suggest a biopsy. And there was a good chance the biopsy would find cancer. Then he'd have to make some hard choices.

Joe replied that a man he'd worked with for years was dying of prostate cancer. Clearly Joe was worried about dying of the disease. Advanced prostate cancer, I agreed, is devastating. This is why the medical profession is desperately trying to find ways of detecting the disease at an earlier stage.

Joe wanted to be assured that if a biopsy revealed cancer and he underwent either surgery or radiation therapy, he would be cured.

"It isn't quite that simple," I replied. "You might be cured of a disease that never would have affected you in the first place."

Although the DRE alone is not a good screening test, I explained that, since he had recently had a normal DRE, any cancer found through screening at this point would probably take a number of years to pose a serious problem for him.

"How many years?"

I shook my head. "That's the sixty-four-thousand-dollar question." I couldn't honestly give him a good answer, but I explained that most early prostate cancer doesn't become life threatening for at least five, and perhaps ten, years.

I briefed Joe on the uncertain natural history of prostate cancer and pointed out the factors weighing against treatment in his case. If we did find prostate cancer, I would be very reluctant to recommend surgery because of his heart condition and emphysema. And if he was treated, he would have to risk the side effects of that treatment.

"But I'll be cured," Joe persisted.

"Probably," I repeated. "But given your age and health, how much more time to enjoy life will that cure give you?" My intention was not to be harsh: I wanted Joe to fully weigh the potential risks and benefits of screening and treatment. He took home several brochures on prostate cancer and its treatment options so that he could discuss his decision with his family.

Ten days later, Joe called. "We've talked it over," he said. "I've decided it's not worth having the PSA test. I'm just going to get on with my life, try to stay as healthy as I can, and enjoy my retirement."

Joe made the decision based on the best information available. Like Joe, many older men who weigh the risks and benefits of the treatment that the PSA might lead to decide to forego screening. This may not necessarily be the best choice, but the decision is based on informed judgment. These men simply favor the quality of their lives over the impact that screening might have on longevity.

Some men say, "If you cannot prove to me that screening and eventual treatment are going to be beneficial in terms of saving my life, then I don't want to start that process at all."

Others make the conscious and educated decision to undergo screening. They fear prostate cancer and the debilitating advanced stages of the disease. They will do whatever they can to diminish this possibility, even if the actual benefit of screening remains scientifically unproven.

How should you answer the tough questions about screening and treatment? The principle of informed consent should be your guide throughout this process. And the detailed discussion of diagnosis and treatment that follows will provide the information you need to make your decisions.

6

Treatment of
Early Prostate Cancer I

The most vexing question you face after a diagnosis of early prostate cancer is, What is the best treatment for me?

You will quickly learn that there is no obvious answer and that several choices are available. Before making decisions about the appropriate treatment, your physician should have as much diagnostic information as reasonably possible. Remember, think of yourself as your doctor's partner in this process. Learning as much as you can about the disease is *your* responsibility.

How the Diagnosis Is Made

Before the development of the PSA test, most men were diagnosed with prostate cancer after undergoing a biopsy because of symptoms of the disease: pain in the lower back, trouble voiding, or the detection of signs of an abnormal prostate during a DRE. Other men underwent TURP surgery for benign prostatic hyperplasia and pathologists detected malignant cells (*see figures 16 and 17*).

Today, the majority of prostate cancer cases are diagnosed after an abnormal PSA level or after an abnormality is detected during a DRE, either of which leads to a biopsy.

In the DRE, the examining physician would believe the gland to be abnormal if it has a suspicious feel, suggestive of prostate cancer. Physicians are trained to differentiate between the typical

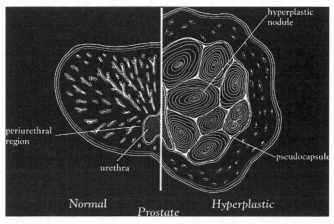

16. Comparative cross-section of healthy and hyperplastic prostates revealing typical BPH involvement
(Courtesy, Merck Human Health Division)

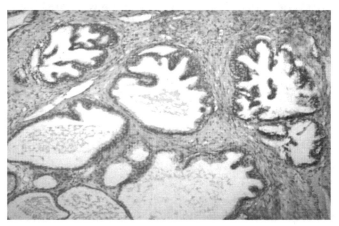

17. Microscopic view of typical BPH in prostate epithelial cells

enlargement and texture of BPH and the equally typical hardening, lumpiness, or palpable nodules of prostate cancer. If your DRE produces such findings, you should undergo a biopsy even if your PSA level is normal. Ask your doctor questions about your DRE results:

- Does my prostate feel enlarged?
- Do you think I have BPH? If so, is it severe?
- Did you feel any hard nodules, lumps, or gritty texture that might suggest prostate cancer?

The Biopsy

Biopsy samples are taken from the suspicious area of the prostate and from other parts of the gland. Usually six small cylindrical samples (called cores) are removed — three from each side of the prostate. Some physicians refer to this procedure as a sextant biopsy.

During the biopsy, the urologist or radiologist usually uses an ultrasonic probe in the rectum to guide a spring-loaded biopsy instrument, or "gun." This probe scans the prostate using high-frequency sound waves, a technique similar to that used to examine a developing fetus in a woman's uterus.

The ultrasonic image of your prostate is displayed on a video monitor to guide the physician's biopsy needle to the proper location. The normal prostate allows sound waves to bounce off it in a uniform fashion. Cancer or BPH change the way the sound waves travel: therefore, an abnormal region often becomes visible. The entire gland is also made visible through ultrasonic image, so your doctor can take representative tissue samples from your prostate.

Ultrasonic imaging reveals suspicious areas of your gland so that a precise biopsy sample can be taken directly from any such site. Also, other tissue samples can be obtained in a representative pattern so that the pathologist can assess whether the cancer resides elsewhere in the gland. Prostate cancer sometimes can be multifocal or patchy, however. Ultrasonic imaging gives an assessment of the gland's size, obvious tumor spread beyond the capsule, and the integrity of the capsule and the seminal vesicles.

During the biopsy, an ultrasonic probe is inserted into the rectum. The procedure is slightly uncomfortable but not actually painful. Each firing of the spring-loaded biopsy gun produces a jab that feels like a hypodermic needle stick. For several days after the biopsy, you may see blood in your urine or ejaculate. Because the biopsy gun pierces the wall of the rectum to extract the samples of prostate tissue, an enema is sometimes given before the biopsy, and oral antibiotics are administered before and after the procedure. There are few significant side effects associated with the prostate biopsy.

The more biopsy material the pathologist is given to examine, the better able he or she is to determine whether cancer is present. The larger the sample, the more conclusive is the establishment of the grade of cancer or how aggressive it appears.

In the past, biopsies were performed manually using a relatively large core sampler, which obtained a significant piece of material for the pathologist to examine. Then the fine-needle aspiration biopsy was developed, in which solid pieces of tissue themselves were not obtained but very small clumps of cells were sucked into the needle to be examined by a pathologist. The results of fine-needle biopsies were often nebulous because of the limited amount of tissue and the absence of a coherent piece of tissue that would reveal the architecture of multiple adjacent cells.

With the advent of the spring-loaded biopsy gun in the 1980s, the procedure was performed faster and with less discomfort. Pathologists now have larger, more structurally consistent samples than those taken from the fine-needle aspiration biopsy. Samples taken by spring-loaded biopsy guns are usually sufficient for recognition of cancer and for Gleason grading.

However, pathologists are occasionally obliged to make important judgment calls based on a biopsy sample that is smaller than they would prefer. In my experience, there is variability among pathologists as they struggle to reach their conclusions on relatively limited material. So the expertise of the pathologist is critical.

Several highly experienced and outspoken American pathologists have defined how gun biopsy samples should be interpreted.

You might show the same sample to different pathologists, though, and get different results. Rarely, however, will one pathologist call a sample cancerous and another will not. More commonly, the grading will be interpreted differently: what is low-grade for one pathologist will be intermediate-grade for another. Again, this variability is based on the often limited amount of biopsy sample available.

The grade of the cancer is critical because it forms one of the most important criteria for your decision on treatment options.

While the criteria are clear for pronouncing a specimen malignant and determining how aggressive a cancer appears, the visual interpretation among pathologists may vary. Pathologists tend to underplay this variability, but it is a significant issue for clinicians and patients who need this information in order to make decisions. This variability will create anxiety. So, without question, if there is disagreement as to whether cancer is present, ask your physician to send the specimen to a pathologist with expertise in prostate cancer. Under such circumstances it may be necessary to obtain a second, independent set of biopsy samples for pathological examination before you and your doctor make decisions on treatment. If there is disagreement about the Gleason score, the grade of the cancer, ask your physician if he or she thinks it prudent for others to examine the samples.

The Diagnostic Role of the PSA

If you have an elevated PSA but a normal DRE, you and your physician must decide whether you should undergo a biopsy. Your doctor might say, "I've scheduled you for a biopsy." Remember that *you* are involved in the decision process. Before deciding on a biopsy, discuss screening fully. The biopsy is a serious step on the diagnostic road to treatment, and, once again, you should participate in this decision based on all the available knowledge.

Keep these important points in mind:

- If your PSA is very elevated — above 10.0 ng/ml — even if the DRE is normal, it is very likely that you have prostate cancer (unless you have prostatitis).
- If your PSA is below 10.0 ng/ml but elevated above the nominal norm of 4.0 ng/ml and your DRE is normal, the likelihood is that you *do not* have prostate cancer. If you do have the disease, however, it is probably in the most curable stage.

Although some physicians will routinely recommend a biopsy, if your PSA is abnormal, there are diagnostic strategies available to determine appropriate candidates for biopsy in order to avoid unnecessary biopsies. These approaches may help you and your physician make the decision about biopsy.

PSA Density

One strategy to determine if you are a candidate for biopsy involves determining what we call your PSA density. This is the prostate-specific antigen value (PSA level in ng/ml) divided by the estimated volume of your gland. The size or volume of your prostate gland is determined by an ultrasound examination, which gives your physician an image of your prostate. Thus, if your PSA is elevated out of proportion to the size of your gland, there is a greater likelihood that you have prostate cancer. If your PSA is elevated only in proportion to (or less than) the size of the gland, as would be seen with BPH, you are less likely to have prostate cancer.

The concept of PSA density as a diagnostic tool comes from our understanding that the level of the PSA protein in your blood is partially related to the size of your gland, which in turn is related to the volume of your prostate epithelial tissue. Further, we know that benign prostatic hyperplasia is a highly prevalent condition. We also know that BPH increases both in prevalence and in actual degree of gland enlargement as men age. Therefore,

PSA density takes into consideration the volume of the gland in any individual.

Medical professionals have touted PSA density as a useful means of separating men with abnormal PSAs into two groups — those who are more likely and those who are less likely to have prostate cancer. PSA density is not infallible, however, because the estimate of the gland's volume is not always accurate. Gland-size calculations based on ultrasound images may be erroneous and can lead to significant misestimates of volume. Also, there is often variability among procedures, depending on the operator and the type of ultrasonic imaging equipment. The PSA density may be a useful adjunct to decision making, but it should not be the sole determinant regarding a biopsy.

Age-Adjusted PSA

Another strategy in determining whether you should undergo a biopsy is to look at your PSA value in relation to your age (which we touched on in Chapter 5). When the range of PSA values was determined several years ago, the normal range was set at 0.0 to 4.0 ng/ml. But this did not take into account the natural increase in PSA with age and growth of the gland. Since the introduction of the test, studies have been conducted to correlate age and PSA levels. We now know for certain that "normal" PSA will increase with age in men who do not have prostate cancer. This research has brought about the concept of age-adjusted PSA values.

Following age-adjusted PSA guidelines, men under 50 might have an *upper normal limit* of 2.5 ng/ml. Under age 60, it might be 3.5 ng/ml. Under 70, it could be 5.5 ng/ml. Above age 70, normal age-adjusted PSA could be as high as 6.5 ng/ml. The evidence is strong enough at this point to consider these new standards when making decisions about biopsies. Remember that the old *normal* limit of 4.0 ng/ml might not be appropriate in your individual case. Specifically, a value of 4.0 ng/ml in a 50-year-old man should prompt further evaluation, but it is normal for the average 70-year-old man. Discuss your PSA in relation to your age with your doctor.

Again, a normal PSA value using either traditional or age-adjusted criteria does not necessarily rule out prostate cancer.

PSA Velocity

Another tool used by some physicians for men with mildly elevated PSA but a normal DRE is PSA velocity. PSA velocity is based on the assumption that levels are more likely to rise rapidly if you have prostate cancer than if you do not. This concept has some merit. In two studies, a series of PSA levels was analyzed during periodic tests over several years both for men who ultimately developed prostate cancer and those who did not. In men who did develop prostate cancer, PSA was seen to increase at a rate greater than 0.8 ng/ml per year. Men without diagnosed prostate cancer undergoing similar periodic PSA tests had rate changes lower than the cancer patients.

On any two successive PSA tests, however, there may be considerable variability, with the level rising or dropping. We don't understand the factors that cause these biologic variables, which may climb sufficiently to precipitate a biopsy. But the cause of the PSA elevation between two tests might *not* be due to a growing cancer. Although PSA velocity is an interesting concept, it does not greatly enhance our ability to discriminate among those men with elevated PSAs who actually have prostate cancer from those who do not. Nonetheless, it's a tool that you and your doctor should be familiar with.

Bound versus Free PSA

Preliminary data suggests that some newer PSA tests that discriminate between different forms of PSA in your blood may help distinguish PSA levels that are elevated due to cancer from those due to BPH, identifying bound and free PSA types. The test is available but definitive studies on its value have not been completed.

Case History: Jeff D.

Last winter I consulted with Jeff D., a 62-year-old self-employed construction engineer. Jeff had not seen a doctor for several years, so he decided that he would treat himself to a full physical examination for his sixtieth birthday. His exam revealed no obvious disease or serious health problems. Jeff requested that the examining internist draw a PSA assay. A few days later he got the results: 5.5 ng/ml.

A meticulous engineer who carefully researched most aspects of his professional and personal life, Jeff had read up on the PSA test. He knew a level below 4.0 ng/ml was normal, and that anything higher was suspicious. "I was convinced then and there I had cancer," he said.

Jeff's doctor informed him that the elevated PSA level might be due to a noncancerous condition, such as benign prostatic hyperplasia, perfectly normal for a man Jeff's age. Jeff was convinced that he had prostate cancer, though. His doctor referred him to a urologist who performed an ultrasonically guided eight-core biopsy of the prostate. On examination by a pathologist, each of the cores was completely negative — free of any microscopic evidence of prostate cancer. Several of the biopsy samples, however, did show BPH, which is what the urologist had suspected.

Jeff remained convinced the biopsy had somehow missed the cancer. Several months later he underwent a second eight-core biopsy. In this biopsy the urologist also took cores from the transition zone of the gland, which borders the urethra, an area that had not been sampled earlier. Again, the results were completely negative. But Jeff's PSA — which he had tested every three months — remained stubbornly elevated, averaging around 5.1 ng/ml.

Something had to be driving up his PSA, Jeff insisted during our consultation. "I probably have a very small cancer that the biopsies missed, don't I?"

We discussed the complexity of the prostate gland — its diseases and conditions and their impact on the PSA test. When Jeff came to me for a consultation, his PSA level had averaged just over 5.0 ng/ml for a year. But a total of sixteen biopsy core samples (including samples from the transition zone) had failed to reveal any indication of cancer. Even after I carefully explained the role BPH and mild but chronic prostatitis plays in long-term elevated PSA, Jeff remained apprehensive, nagged by the worry that undetected cancer lurked in his prostate.

On his second visit, I ordered another ultrasonic imaging of the prostate to more accurately determine the size of Jeff's prostate. The results revealed moderate BPH, a prostate size of 35 grams. This enlargement most likely accounted for his continuing elevated PSA.

After we had the results, we reviewed what we knew about PSA density and velocity. An engineer who was comfortable discussing technical data, Jeff readily grasped the information I presented from the tests and imaging. He understood that there was enough BPH tissue in his prostate to produce his high PSA levels.

"So," he said, smiling broadly for the first time, "I guess I don't have prostate cancer after all."

"Apparently not," I said, returning his smile.

"When should I see you again?"

There really was no reason for Jeff to consult with me again, unless his PSA suddenly shot up and remained high. But I knew he was greatly relieved by the results of the medical tests that proved the absence of a disease or condition.

"Come back in a year," I told him.

Should I Undergo a Biopsy?

As you can see in the case of Jeff D., some physicians advocate performing a biopsy on everyone who has an elevated PSA, even if their digital rectal examination is normal. Is this the correct course for you under similar circumstances? First, make sure that the PSA test has been repeated once or twice to confirm that the level is abnormal. Taking a course of antibiotics to treat the possibility of undetected prostatitis is a reasonable idea. If your PSA remains elevated despite antibiotics, a biopsy should be considered.

Taking a biopsy in every case of elevated PSA is clearly the most aggressive diagnostic approach and would lead to large numbers of men being biopsied (with no cancer being found in the majority).

In general, if you have a long life expectancy and agree to screening with full knowledge and consent, undergoing a biopsy is a good approach. However, some physicians will take into account PSA density, age-adjusted PSAs, and possibly the proportion of free PSA in making a decision about biopsy. Ask your doctor if he or she takes these factors into consideration.

If you undergo a sextant biopsy because of an abnormal DRE or elevated PSA, ample tissue is obtained, and no cancer is found, the evidence strongly suggests that there is no significant cancer in your prostate gland. These biopsies are not absolutely conclusive and you should continue to follow up after the biopsy. However, a good set of negative biopsies should assure you that it is unlikely that you have clinically significant prostate cancer.

After an initial elevated PSA score, subsequent PSA levels may fluctuate or increase. Men in this situation may undergo repeated rounds of biopsies. In some cases the first round of biopsies will not detect cancer but the second one will. If you have multiple negative biopsies over a period of several years, the probability that you have any significant undetected prostate cancer is greatly reduced.

Certain rare individuals have elevated PSAs and cancers that are not in the prostate's peripheral zone (posterior portion) just beneath the capsule. These patients may have an elevated PSA but negative biopsies because the cancerous tissue is in the periurethral area, the transition zone. Therefore, a second round of biopsies should take samples from the transition zone sites, not just the peripheral zones of the lobes.

Points to remember:

- If you have been biopsied because of an abnormal PSA and the pathological findings are negative, you most likely do not have clinically significant prostate cancer.
- If a biopsy reveals pathological evidence of prostate cancer, you should undergo a staging evaluation to determine the extent of the tumor on the Whitmore-Jewett or TNM staging systems.

Staging Evaluation with Bone Scan and CT Scan

The widespread use of scanning tests for staging has become somewhat controversial. In the past, everyone with prostate cancer automatically underwent a bone scan and a CT scan after diagnosis.

The purpose of the bone scan is to determine if there is metastatic spread of prostate cancer to bone or bone marrow (in particular, to the bones of the pelvis, including the hips and the spine, ribs, and legs). When your bone cells are damaged by the growth of metastases, natural tissue repair occurs. The process of bone repair in response to metastatic damage can be seen in a bone scan.

A nuclear medicine physician administers a harmless radioactive isotope marker intravenously, which is absorbed by bone in the process of repair and forms an image that is captured as the density of the radioactivity. A photographic image of your body is then made that can give a reasonably accurate picture of metastatic spread. Although bone turnover (destruction followed by healing) caused by arthritis is also detected in a bone scan, nuclear medicine specialists are trained at distinguishing images of prostate cancer metastasis from noncancer abnormalities.

The computerized tomography (CT) scan is a computer-en-

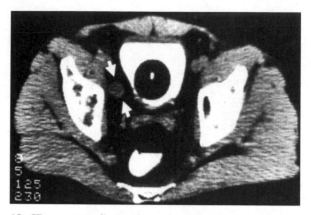

18. CT scan revealing enlarged pelvic lymph node (center, left), indicative of prostate cancer (Courtesy, Merck Human Health Division)

hanced X-ray imaging technique that provides views of horizontal "slices" through your body. The advantage of CT scans over standard X-rays is that they make pictures of your soft, or non-bony, tissue. A CT scan can sometimes yield an image of prostate cancer growth beyond the confines of the gland and of metastatic involvement of your pelvic lymph nodes (*see figure 18*).

With the widespread use of the PSA test, it is becoming increasingly unusual for patients who have recently been diagnosed with prostate cancer to have abnormal CT scans and bone scans (indicative of metastatic disease). Some experts suggest that a bone scan should not be done in somebody with prostate cancer who has a PSA level under 10.0 ng/ml. Studies indicate that the likelihood of a bone scan revealing evidence of metastatic cancer in these people is less than 1 percent (*see figure 19*).

In the past, CT scans were performed more frequently in men with prostate cancer to rule out metastases. Because it is extremely unusual for anyone to have metastases in the lymph nodes if his PSA level is below 20.0 ng/ml and his Gleason score is less than 8, I request a CT scan only for patients who have a PSA level above 20.0 ng/ml or a Gleason score of 8 or above. Under

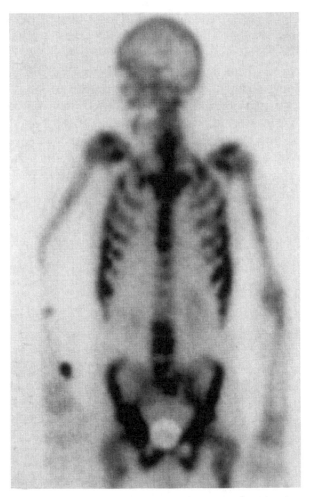

19. Positive bone scan revealing severe metastatic prostate cancer (dark areas) in important bones

specific circumstances, a staging evaluation using both the bone scan and the CT scan is appropriate to determine if you have metastatic prostate cancer.

Each of the scans is specific in its findings. For example, if the bone scan is abnormal and the nuclear medicine physician believes the findings are consistent with metastatic prostate cancer, his diagnosis is generally accurate. A CT scan that shows clear evidence of lymph node enlargement in the pelvis is also convincing evidence of metastatic disease.

Depending on the exact findings of the scans and the degree of suspicion of metastasis, it may be appropriate to perform a biopsy of the suspected metastatic site. During a bone biopsy, a very small portion of bone and bone marrow is removed under local anesthesia. A lymph node biopsy is conducted either in an "open" procedure under general anesthesia or in a "percutaneous" procedure (by needle through the skin after local anesthesia).

Under most circumstances, such a biopsy is not necessary. If a man has a low likelihood of metastatic disease (a low PSA and a low pathological grade in the prostate biopsy sample) but the bone scan appears positive, a biopsy of the site will confirm a diagnosis of metastasis.

In most cases, biopsies of suspected metastases are not necessary. If a patient comes to me with a PSA level of 10.0 ng/ml, a prostate biopsy confirming the presence of cancer, and a positive bone scan, I have enough information to diagnose metastatic prostate cancer. This is based on the extremely high PSA level and the positive bone scan, which is certainly not surprising given this PSA. But let's look at a less obvious case.

Case History: Harold L.

Harold L., a 50-year-old man, had undergone a PSA test that revealed a level of 4.5 ng/ml. Sextant biopsies showed Gleason $3 + 3 = 6$ prostate cancer in one biopsy core. I ordered a bone scan that suggested a metastatic "hot spot" in one of the bones of the pelvis, an area to which prostate cancer typically spreads. An X-ray showed no abnormality. An MRI, which helps detect cancer in bone, was normal. Before I could recommend a radical prostatectomy to Harold, I wanted to make sure that his cancer had not spread. I recommended a bone biopsy, which in Harold's case would be a simple outpatient procedure performed under local anesthesia. Harold's bone biopsy was cancer-free. He had a radical prostatectomy, and he is doing well today.

Endorectal Coil MRI

Another useful diagnostic test that your doctor might recommend is an MRI of the prostate, which involves a rectal probe or coil. This test is similar to an ultrasound of the prostate but gives, I think, better information. I recommend this test for patients who are considering surgery for their cancer and in whom there is possible tumor extension beyond the prostate. Your doctor might want to check an MRI for extracapsular extension or invasion into the neurovascular bundles or seminal vesicles. This means that cancer cells have spread beyond the prostate capsule and are invading the surrounding tissues or the seminal vesicles. If this is the case and the diagnosis is unequivocal, I seldom recommend surgical removal of the prostate as sole treatment.

New Sensitivity for the PSA Test

One of the most important factors in your diagnosis is whether a cancer is contained within your prostate or has spread beyond the confines of the gland. This factor will influence your treatment decision. As we noted earlier, recent research findings offer promise that a new molecular biology technique may help in making complex decisions about appropriate therapy. This technique involves a process called the reverse-transcriptase polymerase chain reaction (RT-PCR) for PSA test.

The RT-PCR is very different from the normal PSA blood test. Bear in mind that every cell in the male body contains the gene capable of producing prostate-specific antigen — and the many other proteins our organs make. But only prostate epithelial cells (normal or malignant) convert that gene's DNA into the messenger chemical we call RNA, which ultimately produces the PSA protein. The RT-PCR test can identify minuscule amounts of this specific RNA messenger chemical. This sensitive test promises to be an important tool in deciding which patients are appropriate for surgery. If you have just been diagnosed with prostate cancer and are undergoing a diagnostic workup, ask your doctor if the RT-PCR test is appropriate in your case.[1] Presently there are too many uncertainties about it to use it to guide treatment decisions.

Questions You Should Ask Your Doctor after Your Diagnostic Workup Is Completed

1. What is your best estimate of the stage of my cancer?
2. Can you explain how you reached this estimate?
3. Can the volume of the tumor be estimated through DRE, biopsy, ultrasound, or MRI? How big is the tumor?
4. Does DRE, ultrasound, or MRI (if performed) suggest any penetration of the prostate capsule?
5. What is your best estimate as to the aggressiveness or metastatic potential of this cancer?

Now that you know how the diagnosis of prostate cancer should be made, how its characteristics are determined, and whether the tumor has spread, we must answer your critical questions.

Should I be treated, and if so, how? To give you a framework within which to understand this complex problem, I address three issues: cure; what your condition would be without treatment; and treatment-associated side effects. I'll discuss these issues in detail in Chapters 7, 8, and 9, but let me introduce them here.

Cure is clearly what you want to achieve, but surprisingly, it can mean two different things. Cure usually means the total eradication of every last cancer cell in your body — a clear concept, and certainly achievable for many patients with prostate cancer. The other definition of cure is more specific to prostate cancer. In this sense cure may not mean wiping out every last cancer cell but rather a sufficient number so that it will never be a problem in your lifetime.

The second issue is how your condition will be affected if you choose not to seek treatment. There are uncertainties, but localized prostate cancer generally does not impact how you will fare over the short term, perhaps for five or more years. However, without treatment, the chances of curing your cancer decrease. Stated another way, your treatment is an investment for the future, perhaps decades from now.

Lastly, remember that any type of treatment will have side effects. You must understand this before moving forward.

Does My Cancer Need to Be Treated?

The question of which types of prostate cancer are significant and which are incidental is a controversial area in medicine. We do not have enough reliable information to suggest inflexible guidelines.

There are men who undergo a prostate evaluation with a PSA and DRE followed by a biopsy — and are diagnosed with prostate cancer — who probably should not have undergone screening in the first place. These might be older men whose realistic life expectancy is ten years or less, or men who suffer from other illnesses who have a realistic life expectancy of only ten years. Several times a month I meet such men with prostate cancer who are anxious to learn what type of therapy is appropriate for them. Another group I am concerned about is younger men whose cancers might not be aggressive and who may never need treatment. Frankly, it is difficult to identify the latter category with any degree of reliability.

Case History: Bob S.

Bob S. is a good example of a patient who does not need treatment. A 78-year-old retired machinist from Rhode Island, he has severe coronary artery disease with unstable angina. The HMO he belongs to routinely orders PSA tests for their male patients over 50. Bob's PSA level was elevated to 7.9 ng/ml and his DRE was normal. He underwent prostate biopsies that revealed cancer in one core from the right side of his gland. The pathological grade of the biopsy sample was moderate, Gleason 6, and a bone scan was negative. I easily concluded that Bob had localized prostate cancer.

When I met Bob in my office, he asked which type of treatment would be best for him. A careful review of his medical records convinced me that he need not undergo any type of aggressive therapy for localized disease. He had no trouble urinating and only slight symptoms of BPH, normal at his age. Bob's life expectancy was shorter than the period of perhaps ten years in which I would reasonably expect this cancer to cause any problem.

I recommended that he choose observation, also known as watchful waiting. (Chapter 8 provides a detailed discussion of watchful waiting.)

Bob is at one extreme of a spectrum of conditions that includes age, overall health, and related life expectancy. Along this spectrum there are also younger men who have cancers that might retain low metastatic potential for the rest of their lives (these are men whose realistic life expectancy might be up to thirty years and who have an extremely low likelihood that their particular cancer will cause a problem during that time). Although we do not have enough data to make firm recommendations about the best course of action in such cases, there is no question that some patients with low-volume, low-grade cancers may not require treatment.[2]

If I've been diagnosed with a type of small, low-grade pros-

tate cancer and I have a life expectancy of twenty or thirty years, which treatment should I seek? Should I opt for watchful waiting?

One drawback to watchful waiting is that there is always some uncertainty about the future behavior of the cancer. For example, did the biopsy truly reflect the volume and the grade of the tumor? Remember that our current level of understanding of low metastatic potential cancers is not perfect. Your doctor may believe that treatment is best for you, erring on the side of caution.

What do I suggest in these tough-call cases? I usually recommend therapy to patients with life expectancies over ten years. I do so for two reasons. First, I do not know how well biopsy samples represent the entire contents of the gland. Second, the natural history of individual prostate cancers is *variable*. Always keep these points in mind as you make your own decision about treatment.

Like many of my patients, you are no doubt anxious if you have been diagnosed with cancer but are not undergoing treatment. It is difficult to hear that you have a malignant prostate tumor that might not require treatment for the rest of your life, and it is particularly difficult to accept this if there are therapies available to treat the cancer.

What I make clear in a postdiagnosis consultation in early prostate cancer cases is that this type of prostate cancer is not an aggressive, rapidly moving malignancy. You have ample time to sort out which treatment options, if any, are appropriate for you, based on your individual needs. Your cancer has most likely existed in your prostate for years and most certainly will not suddenly spread. As a newly diagnosed prostate cancer patient, you certainly have the luxury of weeks to make an informed decision.

Resist the desire to quickly choose a particular treatment option. You've probably lain awake at night thinking *I've got to do something right away to get rid of this damned cancer before it spreads.* But my recommendation is to take as much time as you need to carefully consider the alternatives, even if you are extremely anxious. If your urologist tells you that you may have to wait months for radical prostatectomy surgery unless you agree to have the operation in two weeks, tell the urologist you'll wait, unless you are absolutely ready to make the decision.

Before making a decision, explore all the options and answer all your questions. Many of the issues are controversial, and the situation will be confusing. If you're informed, you'll be better able to participate with your physician in the decision process.

It is often not the man who drives the treatment decision process, but his wife or partner. Your wife might be more objective, more critical, and more inquisitive about your situation than you are. Some men are inclined to obediently proceed in the direction of the first opinion they receive and are often more stoic and trusting in this situation than women. A trusting nature, however, allows you to feel confidence in your physician, and this confidence may give you the resiliency you need to overcome the common side effects of treatment. By all means, though, be a well-informed patient.

Should I Be Treated?

As a newly diagnosed prostate cancer patient whose metastatic workup shows no evidence that the disease has spread beyond the gland, the most important question you need to ask your physician is, If I am treated, what is the likelihood that I will be cured?

The answer to this question is becoming better understood by the medical community. Your physician will consider a number of factors in reaching a decision to recommend treatment. The most important of these factors are the estimated stage, grade, and volume of your cancer, and your PSA level, density, and velocity. Your doctor may also take advantage of new tests, such as the RT-PCR for PSA test.

The second question is, If my cancer is left untreated, what is the likelihood that it will spread and become a problem? This is not easy to answer with any degree of certainty. But the physicians you consult will give you their best educated opinion.

You should ask the following questions:

1. What is the likelihood this cancer will cause a problem five, ten, fifteen, or twenty years from now if it is not treated?
2. What is my likelihood of being cured with surgery, with radiation therapy, and with alternative forms of treatment?
3. If you believe that I have surgically curable (organ-confined) cancer, what is your determination based on?

In answering these questions, your physician should consider your age and overall health. However, it is difficult for your doctor to state conclusively that you won't have to worry about a particular cancer for the rest of your life. And it is not easy to guarantee you'll be cured by treatment. Cure means the cancer will be eradicated. This is distinct from the likelihood of living many years with an untreated — and uncured — cancer.

If the side effects of treatment were trivial, your decision would be easier to make. You could simply proceed with surgery, radiation therapy, or whichever treatment you decided on. In an ideal scenario, the benefits of cure would definitely outweigh the risks of treatment, even if the treatment was not a guarantee of cure. But in the situation that your chance of cure is very low and the risk of side effects is very high, treatment is less desirable. If, however, you choose a treatment with fewer side effects, you gamble that a cure will outweigh the negative factors of treatment — what we call morbidity. I always stress that it is critical to accurately estimate your chance of cure and obtain a clear appraisal of treatment side effects.

Points You Should Consider

1. *Tumor stage.* The most important single factor in staging is the determination of how much of the prostate is occupied by

cancer. The opinion on the extent of the cancer's spread — the tumor stage — is highly subjective: two physicians examining the same gland during a DRE may have a different sense of the cancer's size and whether or not the tumor has extended beyond the confines of the prostate.

The distinction between a stage A and B cancer versus a stage C cancer is critical. This is because we generally regard stage C cancers as incurable. (Remember, your doctor may call stage A and B cancers T1 and T2, and stage C cancer T3.)

Ultrasound and MRI examination of your prostate may distinguish a cancer that has extended beyond the gland (stage C or T3 cancers) from one that is still confined within the prostate.

2. *Cancer grade.* The grade of the cancer — its microscopic appearance to a pathologist — is also relevant to your treatment decision. Most cancers we see are intermediate grade, Gleason 5 through 7. Newly diagnosed cancers in the range of Gleason grade 2 through 4 or grade 8 through 10 are less common.

Gleason grade 2 through 4 cancers have what we call low biological potential: some might never need to be treated. Some fit the category of latent, or autopsy, tumors. Gleason 8 through 10 cancers are usually much more aggressive and are more likely to produce metastases. The biological potential of intermediate grades, Gleason 5 through 7, is hard to determine.[3]

3. *Cancer volume.* The more cancer you have, the greater the chance that the cancer has escaped from your gland. The DRE will help determine the volume of cancer — how much of the prostate feels like normal tissue and how much feels denser and lumpier.

The number of the six or eight biopsy samples that are positive can indicate the extent of the tumor in the gland. If all the specimens show cancer, your tumor is more likely to have a greater volume than if only one core shows cancer.

4. *The tumor's genetic constitution.* The more we learn about prostate cancer, the more tests become available to help us estimate the behavior of a tumor. The tests are designed to clarify the genetic constitution of the tumor. One useful test is called DNA

ploidy.[4] Ask your doctor if this test is appropriate for your diagnostic workup.

5. *PSA.* Your PSA level can help you and your doctor decide on treatment and estimate the probability of cure. As PSA level increases, the chance that a cancer is confined within the prostate decreases. I am concerned about the potential for cure in someone with a PSA level above 15.0 ng/ml. This often indicates cancer beyond the prostate.

Likelihood of Cure

You and your doctor can make a fair estimate of your cure potential when you combine the factors of stage, grade, and volume of the cancer, the PSA, and biologic tests such as DNA ploidy. Though not infallible, this information should help you make a decision about what form of therapy, if any, is appropriate for you.

Remember, the key is to determine the likelihood of cure. Together, you, your family, and the medical professionals you consult can build an informed value system that provides an accurate tradeoff between the likelihood of cure versus the side effects that you may endure following treatment.

This is not an easy issue to consider. I know you do not enjoy pondering your own mortality. And the decision about treatment of prostate cancer has a definite impact on your quality of life. You'll feel better about making such an important decision when you have all the facts.

Case History: Jim D.

Jim D. is 70 years old and has a high-grade cancer (Gleason score 8) and a PSA of 40.0 ng/ml. All six biopsy specimens show grade 8 cancer. But his DRE was surprisingly normal, and his bone scan and CT scan showed no evidence of cancer spread. I told Jim that the prospect that local therapy (surgery or radiation therapy) would cure his cancer was very low, certainly under 50 percent and possibly below 20 percent. This was because the cancer had probably metastasized — although this was not yet apparent in scans.

The fact that the odds are at least 80 percent against a cure is important information: Jim eventually opted for a combination of hormonal and radiation therapies, deciding that surgery was more than he wanted to go through given the low likelihood of cure.

The issues that you will weigh are complex, but your age is certainly important. Jim, recognizing that the chance of cure was low, decided not to have surgery. But a younger man — a 50-year-old, for example — given the same odds might choose the most aggressive therapy and opt for surgery, which would outweigh the negative side effects of treatment.

You should know your realistic life expectancy in order to make the choices that are right for you. If I tell a patient that his chance of cure is low, he might reply, "Then maybe I should opt for no treatment or for the treatment with the fewest side effects." This could be radiation therapy. Or, depending on the individual circumstances, hormone therapy might be more appropriate. I will discuss these treatments in the following chapters.

While some men opt for treatment with the fewest side effects, others say, "Although my chance for a cure is very low, I want to choose the treatment that offers the highest probability of curing this cancer, no matter what the side effects are." In many cases this will be radical prostatectomy. Like Jim, some opt for combination treatments like hormonal therapy followed by radical prostatectomy or by radiation therapy.

None of these options is right or wrong per se. But you should make your treatment decision with as much knowledge as possible. Your physician should reveal all that he or she knows about the nature of your cancer, and then you both should frankly and thoroughly examine your options.

7

Treatment of
Early Prostate Cancer II

Radical Prostatectomy

The purpose of the radical prostatectomy is to cure you of cancer. The operation is best reserved for men who have a high probability of cure (for those who have early prostate cancer). Physicians call the early stage of prostate cancer intracapsular, or organ confined — cancer that has not penetrated the gland capsule and spread to the seminal vesicles or pelvic lymph nodes.

The radical prostatectomy is a procedure that involves the surgical removal of the prostate gland (with the adjacent seminal vesicles) and usually the nearby pelvic lymph nodes. This procedure was introduced earlier this century and has undergone considerable evolution; it is now much safer than it used to be.

Two different surgical techniques, the retropubic and the perineal, are used when performing the radical prostatectomy. The most commonly used technique is the retropubic approach. In this procedure, the surgeon makes an incision in the lower abdomen and removes the pelvic lymph nodes and then the prostate; then the urethra is reattached to the bladder. In the perineal approach, an incision is made in the perineum (the area between the scrotum and the anus). The pelvic lymph nodes are not removed unless a separate abdominal incision is made or a laparoscope is used.

Summary of the Procedure

A radical prostatectomy usually takes between three to five hours and is most often performed under general anesthesia. If epidural anesthesia is used, you are conscious but your lower body is numb. Epidural anesthesia is used if general anesthesia poses a particular risk to you (based on your medical history).

In the retropubic approach, a midline incision is made from below the navel to the pubic bone or a horizontal incision is made above the pubic bone. Usually the surgeons first remove some of the pelvic lymph nodes, and they may wait to continue the procedure while a pathologist examines thin frozen slices of these nodes for evidence of cancer.[1] Many surgeons will proceed with the operation unless the lymph nodes are visibly enlarged with cancer because obvious cancer in the lymph nodes is rarely seen today in radical prostatectomy candidates who have undergone thorough diagnostic workups.

If no cancer is found in the lymph nodes, the surgeons continue with the operation. The prostate and seminal vesicles are surgically separated from the surrounding structures — the bladder, urethra, and rectum. Once separated, the prostate gland is removed by cutting through the urethra beneath the base of the gland, near the external urethral sphincter. The surgeons attach the bladder neck to the urethra, a process that is something like fitting together two sections of garden hose of slightly different diameter. The two ends are attached with multiple fine sutures to produce a urine-tight fit after healing. This suturing is done around a silicone-coated Foley catheter that was earlier inserted into the bladder through the penis. The site where the urethra is sutured and reattached to the bladder neck is called the anastomosis. A reattachment that doesn't leak urine might seem impossible, but it *is* possible.

The Nerve-Sparing Operation

When researching radical prostatectomy and discussing it with your doctor, you're sure to hear about the nerve-sparing procedure developed by Dr. Patrick Walsh of Johns Hopkins University. His technique revolutionized the way the operation is performed.

The principle behind the nerve-sparing procedure is to clamp and suture the blood vessels so that the surgical team can see the fine details of the prostate and surrounding structures. Able to see the structures clearly, the surgeon can better identify the extent of disease before the prostate is removed. In this procedure the surgeon works carefully to dissect the prostate from the surrounding structures, most importantly, from the two neurovascular bundles, a fine network of nerves and blood vessels on the gland's outer capsule. The surgeon can spare the nerves that are critical to the ability to achieve erection. In the past, radical prostatectomy invariably severed these nerves during the removal of the gland because surgeons could not see them clearly enough to permit fine dissection. This resulted in complete impotence following radical prostatectomy.

The paired neurovascular bundles, which look like thin strings with feathery threads attached, adhere directly to the outer surface of the prostate gland. By leaving the neurovascular bundles intact, Dr. Walsh aimed to preserve sexual function in his patients.

Although the nerves can be spared in this technique, the preservation of sexual potency is not guaranteed. In fact, many men who undergo this procedure still lose the ability to have erections sufficient for intercourse. Younger men generally have the greatest chance for maintaining potency with the procedure. Furthermore, since the 1980s, surgeons are more reluctant to perform the nerve-sparing procedure because, in sparing one or both neurovascular bundles, they may fail to remove adjacent cancerous prostate tissue. Picture again a series of threads glued to the skin of an apple: it is very difficult to separate them without also taking some of the apple to which they are attached.

An attempt to preserve the nerves should be an option for some patients. If you are potent to begin with, ask your doctor if your cancer is clearly confined to a part of the prostate that is well removed from the outer capsule and the nerve bundles. If it is not confined to that section of the prostate, the nerve-sparing radical prostatectomy is not a viable option for you.[2]

Biopsy of the Lymph Nodes

Let's expand briefly on the purpose of the pelvic lymph node biopsy. The removal of these lymph nodes does not treat the prostate cancer, but allows the surgeon to check for the presence of cancer cells in order to determine if the cancer has spread beyond the gland. During the biopsy the excised nodes are frozen with liquid nitrogen; then thin slices are shaved off for inspection under the microscope. The biopsy normally takes less than thirty minutes.

If the surgeon does not strongly suspect spread to the lymph nodes, he may proceed without obtaining frozen section results. These days, spread of cancer to the lymph nodes is very unusual and is discovered in fewer than 10 percent of prostatectomy procedures. This is no doubt due to the early detection strategies now being employed.[3]

Discovery of prostate cancer in your pelvic lymph nodes indicates that the cancer has spread to the lymph system and very likely to other parts of your body. Lymph node biopsy during prostatectomy is similar to the removal of axillary lymph nodes in the underarm during breast cancer surgery in order to stage the cancer and assess the possible metastatic spread of the disease.

Cancer that involves the pelvic lymph nodes is classified as stage D1 disease. This is distinct from stage D2, which signifies detectable spread to bone or other areas of the body. Most urologists would not continue with the radical prostatectomy if the lymph nodes were obviously swollen with cancer because it doesn't make much sense to remove the prostate after the disease has escaped from the gland. Remember, the purpose of the radical prostatectomy is to totally eradicate the cancer from your body. Once the cancer has spread to the lymph nodes, it most likely has spread elsewhere, and the benefit of removing the prostate gland is uncertain.

If you choose radical prostatectomy, you'll undoubtedly be advised before undergoing surgery that if cancer is found in your pelvic lymph nodes, your cancerous prostate will not be removed.

Immediate Postoperative Care

You most likely will remain in the hospital for three to five days following a radical prostatectomy. You'll be up and around fairly quickly because postoperative pain is minimized through the use of analgesics, including narcotics. Do not be too worried about the painful aftermath of this surgery. You also will be able to eat within a few days.

The Foley catheter that was placed in your bladder during surgery will remain there after you return home, usually for three weeks. This allows the reattached urethra time to heal. Expect to be recuperating at home (but not bedridden) for ten days to three weeks.

Urinary Incontinence

Urinary incontinence is one of the potential unpleasant side effects of the radical prostatectomy surgery. The external urethral sphincter is disrupted by the severing of the urethra at the base of the bladder and the reattachment of the bladder neck to the urethral stump below the site of the removed prostate. Unfortunately, the internal urethral sphincter that provides involuntary urine control is usually lost or scarred as a result of surgery.

Following surgery, you may experience varying degrees of difficulty in your ability to control your urine. At first, after the catheter is removed, most men do not have normal control over their urine; the sphincter has to be retrained to control a different type of urethra.

Your doctor may recommend a series of Kegel exercises that strengthen your pelvic muscles. Kegel exercises are performed by repeatedly flexing and relaxing the muscles that stop the urine stream (the muscles that tighten the urinary and rectal sphincters). Kegel exercises can improve the tone of the cylindrical muscles of the external urethral sphincter. The improved tone and strength of the sphincter greatly enhance control of urine.

Some men gain almost complete control of their urine as soon as the catheter is removed; others take weeks or months to regain continence. Others have persistent urinary incontinence of varying degrees, which is similar to the stress incontinence experienced by some women in later life. This is caused by physical exertion of some type, such as sneezing, lifting a heavy weight, or swinging a golf club or tennis racket. Stress incontinence is not a complete loss of urinary control, but rather a leakage that often requires the use of a urine-absorbing pad. Several manufacturers also produce underwear made of extra-absorbent material. Moderate your intake of alcohol; alcohol tends to relax the sphincter and may temporarily exacerbate the problem.

It's rare that a man has complete, permanent urinary incontinence following surgery. Most men retain reasonable control over their urine, but others require a pad. This condition often improves over time.[4]

Dr. James Talcott, a member of our group studying the prevalence of urinary incontinence following radical prostatectomy, found that one year after surgery:

- 35 percent of the men studied wore an underwear pad to protect against stress incontinence and urine dribble.

- 11 percent had regular moderate stress incontinence.
- Most patients had regained complete control of their urine one year after radical prostatectomy.

Discuss any prolonged urinary incontinence problems after radical prostatectomy with your doctor. The Kegel exercises should help a little. Make sure you are exercising correctly; your doctor or physical therapist should be able to help. We'll discuss this problem in greater detail in Chapter 9.

Another type of urinary problem may occur months after surgery: a bladder neck contracture, or a urethral stricture. Although unusual, this is caused by excess scar tissue that may form after the surgery. If your urine flow is slowed or it is difficult to urinate, this may be the reason. Bring the problem to your doctor's attention; a simple operation can correct it.

Sexual Function after Surgery

Your libido, or sex drive, is generally controlled by your hormones. In no way does the radical prostatectomy alter the hormonal control of sexual desire. After prostate cancer surgery, you should maintain normal levels of the male hormone testosterone, which is mostly produced in your testes. So, from a hormonal standpoint, radical prostatectomy does not change your prior level of sex drive.

A man's ability to achieve erection is almost always affected by surgery. Penile erection is a complex process that is controlled in part by the nerves that surround the prostate. However, erectile function depends on factors other than input from these nerves, and many men become impotent even when both sets of nerves are spared during a prostatectomy.

After radical prostatectomy, you might be able to achieve orgasm but not a full erection. This is because the nerves involved in orgasm are separate from the neurovascular bundles that control erection. The volume of your ejaculated semen is also significantly diminished or absent because, without a prostate or seminal vesicles, the principal sources of your semen are gone.

Dr. Talcott further found that the chances of sexual dysfunction are (including impotence) following radical prostatectomy. One year after surgery:

- 75 percent of men studied had not had an erection in the four weeks prior to polling.
- Only 7 percent had had erections adequate for intercourse.

You and your partner should both understand that there is a high probability that your ability to achieve an erection will be affected by surgery no matter what type of procedure is used and no matter who the surgeon is. Even with the nerve-sparing operation, the likelihood that you will easily achieve erections adequate for intercourse is quite low.[5] I would advise the nerve-sparing procedure to a highly select group of relatively young patients who have strong erections before surgery and whose cancers are small and organ confined.

Because surgeons are concerned that the nerve-sparing prostatectomy fails to preserve sexual function, some have adopted the policy of not sparing the nerves and, with their patient's consent, inserting an implanted penile prosthesis during the procedure. This approach, which we'll discuss in Chapter 9, may be attractive for certain men.

Radical Prostatectomy and Cure Potential

Remember, the purpose of the radical prostatectomy is to completely remove the tumor from the body. The pathologist determines whether this has been accomplished by analyzing the surgically removed prostate gland and lymph nodes for the presence of cancer.

The pathologist must learn whether or not the cancer was completely contained within the gland — that all malignant tissue was confined within the capsule surrounding the prostate. For the pathologist, this is relatively straightforward; examination of the surgically removed prostate readily reveals the extent of tumor involvement. In many cases the cancer is clearly confined to the gland, with no evidence of growth of tumor beyond the prostate.

The pathologist will microscopically examine the architecture of the tumor to determine the grade of malignancy with a Gleason score. High-grade cancers (Gleason 8 through 10) have a higher likelihood of recurring — due to preoperative spread — even if the cancer appears to be confined within the gland.

A cancer that is not confined within the prostate capsule may be apparent in various ways and with different implications. Cancer can grow through the capsule, with tumor tissue extending beyond the normal confines of the gland into the surrounding tissues of your pelvic cavity. In a similar manner, the pathologist might learn that the margins of your prostate — the edges of the specimen which were cut when it was removed from the surrounding structure — contain malignant cells, implying the presence of remaining cancer cells. The pathologist might also find that your seminal vesicles, which are connected to your prostate, contain cancer. And combinations of these conditions can exist.

The best news your doctors can tell you after surgery is that the malignant tumor tissue was not high-grade and was completely contained within the capsule of the prostate gland. This means the likelihood of your long-term survival and cure is quite high. But if the capsule, the seminal vesicles, or the surgical margins of your prostate have been invaded by cancer, your likelihood of cure is diminished. Cancer in the capsule alone but not in the surgical margins of your prostate implies that the cancer may recur; however, there is significantly more risk of this if the cancer has spread to the surgical margins or the seminal vesicles.

When a pathologist discovers cancer in the surgical margins, the margins are said to be positive. There is considerable controversy about the implication of positive margins in prostate cancer. In breast or colon cancer, positive margins mean that all of the cancer was not surgically removed.

In the case of prostate cancer, positive margins usually mean that some cancer cells were left behind, usually because the cancer was slightly more extensive than had been anticipated preoperatively. Even if the surgeon believes he has removed the entire tumor, the pathologist might find microscopic evidence that cancer extends beyond the excised tissue. Talk to your doctor frankly about this situation. As we will discuss, under certain circumstances, radiation treatment following surgery may eradicate the remaining cells.

Generally, if the pathological examination reveals that your cancer was organ confined, there is no need for further therapy. In this case we can say with great likelihood that your cancer has been cured.

Non-Organ-Confined Disease: Treatment Options

If the pathologist finds that the cancer has extended through your prostate capsule to the margins or to your seminal vesicles, you will decide whether you should receive further therapy. Here we must rely more heavily on scientific and medical principles than on hard data from research studies.

The risk of recurrence through metastasis is highest for seminal vesicle involvement, lower for positive margins, and lower still if there is simple capsule penetration. Most patients with seminal vesicle involvement will have disease recurrence, while probably less than 50 percent of those with simple capsular penetration will.

Radiation therapy is an option if the cancer has spread to the surgical margins, in which case radiation may be curative. Radiation may also be used if the lymph nodes or the seminal vesicles are involved. In such cases the radiation will not likely cure the cancer. Hormonal therapy (see Chapter 8) may be used as well, and we will discuss this in greater detail in Chapter 10. The level of PSA in your blood following surgery will play a crucial role in your decision to undergo further treatment. To know where you stand after surgery, ask the following questions:

Questions to Ask Following Radical Prostatectomy

1. What did the pathologist find? How much of the gland was involved with cancer?
2. Was the cancer confined to the gland?
3. Has the cancer penetrated my prostate capsule? Are my margins positive; are my seminal vesicles involved; are my lymph nodes involved?
4. What is my exact pathological stage and grade of cancer?
5. Based on all this information, what is my likelihood of cure?

Radical Prostatectomy: Conclusions

Physicians call the radical prostatectomy the gold standard of treatment. The radical prostatectomy has the best potential for cure if your cancer is contained within the confines of your prostate gland — the likelihood of cure in such cases is very high. If surgery reveals that the tumor is confined to your prostate, you are very likely to be spared the possibility that cancer cells have escaped. The cure potential for organ-confined prostate cancer coupled with the knowledge that the cancer has been removed make the radical prostatectomy the gold standard. Keep this in mind as you consider your treatment options.

The side effects of surgery, however — especially impotence and incontinence — are difficult to accept, particularly if you have reason to believe that your tumor might not be life threatening if left untreated. Therefore, I reserve the radical prostatectomy for certain types of patients — men who have a high likelihood of being cured by the procedure and also need to be treated due to the aggressive nature of their tumor coupled with an anticipated long life expectancy. Further, these surgery candidates should have a realistic understanding of the treatment-related side effects and be willing to undergo the treatment in an attempt to be cured.

Dr. Willet F. Whitmore, Jr., former chief of urology at Memorial Sloan-Kettering Cancer Center, stated this philosophical position very clearly in the *Journal of the American Medical Association* in 1993: "It is indisputable that aggressive therapy is unnecessary for some and insufficient for others, but the possibility that it may be both necessary and sufficient for a currently undefined subset of patients provides an arguable basis for its use."

Dr. Whitmore knew whereof he spoke. In the mid-1980s, at the age of 68, he was diagnosed with prostate cancer. He chose not to be aggressively treated. Willet Whitmore eventually died of prostate cancer in May 1995 at the age of 78. He enjoyed a good quality of life for most of the years of postdiagnosis survival.

Preoperative Hormone Therapy: "Downstaging" or "Neoadjuvant Hormone Therapy"

An option that your physician may suggest and which you may hear about at support groups is preoperative hormonal therapy, often called downstaging or neoadjuvant hormone therapy. The patient receives treatment for several months prior to surgery to reduce the size of the tumor, enabling the surgeon to better remove the cancer in its entirety. One randomized study (in which about one half of the patients receive one form of therapy and the other half receive another therapy) indicated that preoperative hormonal therapy reduced the rate of positive margins (cancer not completely removed in the surgery).

Several questions remain unanswered, however. These include what type of hormonal therapy to use and what the duration of treatment should be. The most important question is whether this form of treatment will increase your likelihood of cure. Will the use of hormonal therapy at this time decrease the effectiveness of hormonal treatment at a later time? I am cautious about this approach, for though it is possible you will benefit from preoperative hormonal downstaging, it is unproven. Hormonal treatment does have side effects (see Chapter 10). This approach does have the potential of subjecting greater numbers of men to unnecessary aggressive treatment; in addition, it may alter the ability of the pathologist to interpret your postoperative pathologic specimen and thereby change your physicians' recommendations after surgery. If you are willing to accept these risks, discuss this approach with your doctor.

Case History: Successful Radical Prostatectomy

Paul W. is a 66-year-old retired teacher who taught carpentry and metalworking in Boston public schools for forty years. His retirement health insurance is administered through a suburban HMO. During a routine physical examination, Paul's physician performed a DRE. The doctor felt a nodule on the left lobe of the prostate and took a PSA test.

Paul's PSA level was high, 8.0 ng/ml. This was suspicious, even for a man who was 66 and had a history of moderate benign prostatic hyperplasia. One of the HMO's urologists conducted a sextant biopsy. A week later, Paul learned the results: two of the six biopsy cores were positive for prostate cancer. The pathological findings revealed a Gleason score of 3 + 3, a moderately aggressive tumor that was apparently confined to the upper portion of the left side of Paul's prostate. His bone scan was normal, showing no evidence of metastasis.

Two weeks after the biopsy, Paul and his wife, Rose, came to my clinic for a consultation. Like other couples I have consulted, they were afraid of possible imminent death from prostate cancer. I assured them that Paul's tumor appeared only moderately aggressive. And, as Paul was in overall good health, his life expectancy was probably more than ten years. Therefore, I suggested he consider either radiation therapy or radical prostatectomy, both of which would offer a good chance of cure.

Paul wanted to know which treatment was better. He asked, "Which treatment will definitely get rid of the prostate tumor?" He didn't want any cancer left in his body. Paul's wife nodded vigorously as he spoke. They had discussed this issue and decided that the most definitive treatment available — regardless of side effects — would bring them both optimal peace of mind.

I explained that the radical prostatectomy is the current gold standard of curative treatment, the procedure to which all other treatments should be compared. I added that radiation therapy would be a reasonable alternative, as it was less disruptive for a person his age.

Paul shook his head stubbornly. "I'm pretty tough, Doctor," he said.

Indeed, he was in good shape and had no overt signs of cardiovascular disease or pulmonary problems. Paul was probably in as good condition as many men ten years younger; thus he was an appropriate candidate for surgery, if that was his preference. I explained the side effects, including some incontinence during the first postsurgical year and probable permanent sexual dysfunction. Paul and Rose said they knew that sexual impotence could be treated. They had done their homework.

I outlined the treatment options for sexual dysfunction, including the vacuum device and injected medications (see Chapter 9). "We'll handle that if we have to," Paul said.

Paul underwent radical prostatectomy last June. The postsurgical pathological examination revealed the prostate cancer was indeed organ confined and mainly limited to the upper aspect of the left lobe's peripheral zone. There was no capsule penetration, no involvement of seminal vesicles, and no positive surgical margins. The excised pelvic lymph nodes were entirely free of cancer.

Paul had a relatively normal recovery period. His postsurgical incontinence was more troubling than he had anticipated. He consulted his urologist, who discovered Paul was not correctly practicing the recommended regimen of Kegel exercises. The problem was corrected, and Paul's urinary control returned almost completely over several months. After consulting his urologist, Paul obtained a vacuum device and received instructions in the use of injected penile medications to overcome sexual dysfunction.

Soon after surgery, Paul's PSA had dropped to undetectable levels, a good indication that he was cured of prostate cancer.

Case History: An Unusually Rapid Recovery

General H. Norman Schwarzkopf is one of the best known Americans to have recently undergone treatment for prostate cancer. His story is becoming more typical as widespread PSA screening has increased awareness of prostate cancer in the medical community.

In 1994, General Schwarzkopf visited a Florida hospital near his home to have tendinitis in a knee treated. While there, he visited the urology department to discuss the urinary problems he was having. Schwarzkopf later told a *Washington Post* health reporter, "Late in the evening, I would find that I had a strong urge to urinate."

As a retired United States Army general, Schwarzkopf underwent annual physical examinations at military or V.A. hospitals. He knew his most recent PSA level, 1.2 ng/ml, was perfectly normal for a healthy man of 59. A urologist at the hospital took blood for additional tests and performed a thorough DRE. During the rectal examination, the urologist detected a suspiciously hard area. Schwarzkopf's PSA level had risen marginally to 1.8 ng/ml, still within the normal limit. The urologist scheduled a sextant biopsy.

When Schwarzkopf heard the results of the pathological examination, he was flabbergasted. "My brain was just reeling," he said.

The biopsy had detected an apparently small, low-grade prostate cancer.

Schwarzkopf considered all his options. Given the apparent low volume and pathologically confirmed low grade of the tumor, observation or watchful waiting was one of his options, as was radiation therapy or radical prostatectomy. He quickly ruled out observation. "I don't think that anyone with a type A personality could have cancer growing in you and get tested every quarter. What a terrible way to live," he added. In this regard, Schwarzkopf voiced the anxiety felt by many men in his situation. "I wanted to get rid of it."

After carefully considering radiation therapy, both external beam and implant, he weighed the option of cryosurgery. Schwarzkopf found the ambiguity of cure with external radiation therapy intolerable. He also found the still-experimental nature of implant radiation and cryosurgery unacceptable. This left radical prostatectomy. "But once I decided what my course of action was," Schwarzkopf said, "I wanted to make damn sure I got a second opinion."

Schwarzkopf opted for surgery at Walter Reed Army Medical Center in Washington. He also elected the nerve-sparing procedure, should his surgeon determine it was appropriate during the course of the operation.

Schwarzkopf was operated on in May 1994. Hours after the operation, he was walking the hospital corridors, pulling his Foley catheter. A week later, he began to walk the long circular driveway of his home. Within ten days, he had increased his daily walking regimen to five miles.

"I was convinced that if I could get my muscle tone back," he later explained, "my body would function normally."

Indeed, after the catheter was removed two weeks after surgery, Schwarzkopf experienced no incontinence whatsoever, a tribute to both his surgeon's skill and his own iron will.

Even though he had undergone the nerve-sparing procedure, Schwarzkopf did concede that impotence became a problem. However, he stated he had begun using standard techniques to alleviate sexual dysfunction.

Only five weeks after undergoing the radical prostatectomy, Schwarzkopf was waist deep in an icy Alaskan river, salmon fishing with his son. Later that year, he took a four-week photo safari in Africa. In 1995 Schwarzkopf told the *Washington Post*, "Life has returned to normal."

8

Treatment of
Early Prostate Cancer III

Radiation Therapy and Other Nonsurgical Treatments

Radiation therapy is an important treatment option for early prostate cancer. It differs from the radical prostatectomy in that there is no surgical procedure. The prostate is not removed. With standard external-beam radiation therapy, radiation kills cancer cells in place. In general, the negative side effects, what your doctors might call the morbidity of treatment, are less severe than those of the radical prostatectomy.

Radiation therapy has been an important weapon in the fight against cancer for many years. Shortly after the discovery of radium in 1895, doctors learned that malignant tumors would shrink after exposure to radiation. The first prostate cancer patients to receive radiation therapy had pellets of radium inserted in their urethras.

The radiation therapy you receive today destroys the cancer cells in your body by affecting their ability to reproduce or by stimulating a biochemical self-destruction process called apoptosis. Some cancers, like Hodgkin's disease or testicular cancer, are very sensitive to radiation treatment. Other cancers, like melanoma of the skin, are resistant to radiation, even in high doses. Prostate cancer is somewhere in the middle.

In the 1940s and 1950s, moderate-energy X-ray units and cobalt 60 radiation emitters were introduced. They deliver "external beam" (or directed energy) therapy. Radiation equipment has evolved steadily in recent decades. Today the standard prostate cancer treatment is external-beam radiation, given with deep-penetrating, high-energy X-rays that are generated from a machine called a linear accelerator.

If you choose external-beam radiation therapy — sometimes called radical radiotherapy — there are several important factors to keep in mind. The key people treating you are the radiation oncologist (a physician trained in radiation cancer treatment), the physicists who help plan the radiation field, and the technicians who assist in both the planning and the treatment process.

Radiation therapy must be administered with great precision. The key to successful treatment is the skill of the key personnel in assuring that the radiation dosage is optimized to the prostate and minimized to the surrounding normal tissues.

Traditionally, clinicians approximated the position of the prostate by injecting dye into the bladder and rectum. Today, more precise scanning techniques better locate the prostate so that the radiation beam can be precisely aimed. Modern radiation therapy uses computers to visualize the prostate at the intersection of three planes. This is called the simulation, or planning, for radiation therapy.

The most impressive technical advance in external-beam radiation therapy is a recently introduced technology called three-dimensional conformal radiation. During this technique you undergo a radiation-therapy planning CT scan as you lie on a table beneath a large, movable, overhead beam emitter. Your internal image is transferred to a radiation therapy computer and then reconstructed to form a 3-D picture of your prostate and seminal vesicles (the radiation target), as well as the important adjacent normal tissue structures (the bladder and rectum).

Three-dimensional conformal radiation allows precise beaming of radiation fields. Because the exact location of the prostate is more certain, the radiation therapist can also use larger lead-shielding blocks at the radiation beam aperture to narrowly focus the beam and thus protect noncancerous body structures. "Conformal therapy" was so named for these lead blocks, which conform to the shape of the prostate and seminal vesicles. This may prove to be a good upgrade over earlier forms of radiation therapy, in which a larger area of healthy tissue in the lower pelvis was irradiated, producing considerable side effects. Research is under way to plan 3-D radiation using the MRI, which enables even better visualization of the prostate than does the CT scan.

In considering radiation therapy for prostate cancer, ask if conformal external-beam treatment is appropriate for you and is available in your area. If it is not, you may want to locate a cancer treatment center that does provide this type of treatment. If travel is not practical, ask your radiation oncologist what form of simulation is used to precisely target your prostate and to locate your surrounding noncancerous structures. You are entitled to the best planning strategy available.

Before treatment, ask your radiation oncologist:

- If conformal radiation is available, is the equipment up-to-date?
- What type of simulation do you use to locate the prostate and surrounding structures?

The Treatment Course

If you choose to undergo radiation therapy, you will most likely receive treatment in the radiation department of the hospital. After changing into a gown, you will lie on the treatment table underneath the linear accelerator. The treatment technician or therapist carefully positions you, makes sure the lead beam-focusing blocks are in place, and then activates the radiation beam. You might hear a brief, low buzz, but you'll feel no heat or pain. You can expect treatment to last for about five minutes per day. Your treatments are given five times a week, with weekends off.

The course of your treatment continues for seven or eight weeks, involving approximately thirty-five to forty sessions. During the first five weeks of therapy, a slightly larger area is treated, followed by a "cone down" (a more tightly focused radiation field) in the last two to three weeks.

Your predetermined radiation field is controlled by the therapist and by several computers that constantly monitor the treatment parameters, especially the width of the radiation beam. The linear accelerator automatically shuts off when your desired treatment dose is achieved.

Side effects from radiation may occur during treatment or weeks, months, or years afterward. However, external-beam radiation therapy is generally easier to endure than radical prostatectomy.

Short-term side effects are those that occur during or immediately after your radiation therapy. During the treatment you might experience fatigue, but you can usually continue working and carrying out your daily activities. Other short-term side effects include urinary urgency and frequency, usually caused by irritation of the bladder. You also might have slight rectal discomfort and more frequent bowel movements during your treatment. The bladder irritation generally does not require medical intervention and will subside a few weeks after you complete radiation therapy. Medication might be prescribed, which is helpful. The effect on bowels subsides, but this may take months. Severe prolonged problems are rare, but some men experience a change in the number of their bowel movements per day and sometimes have mucous in the stool for many months or years.

Long-term side effects are those that you might experience months after your treatment has ended. The most important is sexual dysfunction, which occurs in most men who were sexually active prior to therapy. Research studies indicate that one year after external-beam radiation, men have about a 50 percent risk of being unable to spontaneously achieve an erection adequate for intercourse. Unfortunately, after radiation therapy the rate of

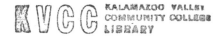

sexual problems increases with time. After two years, most men are impotent.

After radiation therapy, you may experience urethral strictures similar to those that occur after radical prostatectomy. If urinating becomes increasingly difficult months after treatment, do tell your doctor.

Implant Radiation Therapy (Brachytherapy or Interstitial Radiation)

Radioactive implants are small radioactive "seeds" that are inserted into the prostate, placing the radiation source close to the cancerous cells of the tumor. These implants produce principally particle radiation that does not penetrate tissue as deeply as the high-energy X-rays and gamma rays generated in external-beam radiation. The seeds emit radiation for weeks until all the radiation has decayed. Implants have long been used with success in the treatment of other types of cancer.

Until recently, physicians were leery of radiation implants because they were tried with mixed success years ago. In the past, radiation oncologists or urologists were not able to precisely implant the radioactive seeds in the prostate. If the seeds were too close together, "hot spots" would occur, with possible overdosing to normal surrounding tissue. If the seeds were too far apart, "cold spots" occurred, thus undertreating the cancer. Today, computerized scanning and implant-guiding methods permit more precise delivery of the seeds into the cancerous prostate tissue. As a result, implants are making a comeback in the United States. The most commonly used seeds are those made of radioactive palladium or gold.

If you opt for implants, the metallic radiation seeds are usually inserted by the urologist or radiation oncologist through the skin of the perineum (the area between the scrotum and rectum). The physician guides the seeds into the prostate under visualization of the gland by CT scan or ultrasound. A technique is being developed to place seeds using MRI, which may allow more precision. The potential advantage of seed implants is that they deliver radiation to the tumor and minimize radiation to surrounding tissue. With good planning, more radiation can be delivered to the tumor than that which is given by external-beam radiation. At some centers, seeds are being used in conjunction with external-beam radiation with the hope that more radiation can be delivered to the prostate. In my mind, the jury is still out on the use of implants with or without external-beam radiation. The long-term curative effect of implants on prostate cancers is still unknown, but the results after slightly more than five years appear promising.

Implant radiation therapy might well prove to be a reasonable treatment option, particularly for smaller cancers in small glands (less than 60 grams). The proponents of radiation implants believe it minimizes the side effect of sexual dysfunction. Although discomfort with urination and an urgency to urinate are common and may persist for months after implantation, urinary incontinence is rare. These are the reasons the man in our first case history, Bill J., opted for implants. However, rectal injury as a side effect of implants may occur more frequently than with external-beam radiation, although improvements are being made to minimize this side effect.

If you choose this option, I strongly advise you to go to a center that has extensive experience with it. Ask the staff at the center these questions:

- How long have you been performing implant therapy?
- Do you use ultrasound, CT, or MRI scanning to guide implant placement?
- What have the results been at this center to date?

Radiation Therapy: The Curative Potential

Do you have as good a chance of being cured with external-beam radiation therapy (EBRT) as with radical prostatectomy? There is no simple answer to this crucial question. No research directly comparing the principal forms of therapy for prostate cancer — surgery, radiation therapy, and watchful waiting — has been conducted. So, in the absence of good comparative data, you will have to rely on the following general observations about the curative potential of the different treatments.

- Patients who currently undergo EBRT tend to be older and more frequently have another illness, such as cardiovascular disease, than men who receive surgical therapy.
- Men who receive EBRT tend to have more advanced prostate cancer. Often their physicians suspect that since the cancer has probably spread locally in the pelvis, surgery is not an appropriate treatment.
- In general, men treated with EBRT tend to have signs or symptoms of more advanced cancer or to be older than those who undergo surgery, making direct comparisons difficult. Therefore, comparing the results of surgery and radiation is like comparing apples and oranges.
- The effectiveness of EBRT, like that of other treatments, depends to a large degree on the aggressiveness of a cancer and on the extent to which cancer cells have spread prior to treatment. There is controversy regarding the effectiveness of radiation therapy in completely eradicating a prostate cancer.

With this in mind, many doctors understand that radiation works for some, but not all, patients. For some men undergoing radiation therapy, the cancer may be fully eradicated. In others, the cancer may be significantly reduced. The reduction of your cancer by radiation therapy may be sufficient for you to control prostate cancer for five, ten, or even fifteen years. This is a major benefit if your life expectancy could be compromised by untreated prostate cancer.

In some men, the cancer is not eradicated by radiation therapy and it eventually metastasizes, despite the treatment. And in some men, metastasis has occurred before treatment. These men will ultimately display metastasis no matter what form of local therapy is used. Such men have undetected metastases at the time of radiation. Others who receive radiation but eventually suffer cancer recurrence have tumor cells that are resistant to radiation. There is a debate raging as to whether these patients represent a small or a large fraction of men treated by radiation.

Here are some thoughts about radiation therapy that you should consider:

- The majority of patients derive benefit from EBRT either because they are cured by radiation or their disease is retarded long enough so that they do not suffer significant disease before the end of their lives.
- The number of men who could have been cured by surgery but instead opt for radiation, then go on to develop incurable metastatic disease is relatively small.
- Radiation is probably better therapy for smaller tumors than larger ones. Remember, a large prostate tumor that extends into the surgical margins after prostatectomy is a potential problem as well.
- Large tumors contain a larger number of cancer cells and it is difficult for radiation to kill every last cell in these tumors.
- We don't yet have enough research data to predict with great accuracy those patients who will not be cured with radiation.

There are some men for whom radiation therapy will be curative — all their cancer cells will be killed. Other men will achieve a remission — their cancer will cause no problem — but no cure. This remission of disease, however, may be enough for you to enjoy a normal life.

If you are young with a long life expectancy, you should be more cautious about EBRT. Although radiation will cure some patients, it may not eradicate all the cancer cells from some of these men for the rest of their lives. So, if you are a younger

man who has been diagnosed with organ-confined cancer, surgery — despite its side effects — might be your best form of
treatment.

Case History: Ambiguous Prognosis

Dan O. is fighting prostate cancer with energy and spirit. He is an
active salesman in the New England defense electronics industry
who travels widely around the region and has achieved substantial professional success. In June 1993, at the age of 49, Dan
underwent a physical that included a PSA assay. His PSA was
very high: over 35.0 ng/ml.

The DRE was abnormal and a sextant biopsy showed evidence
of prostate cancer. Ultrasonic imaging and DRE suggested a significant tumor in the right side of the gland. The Gleason score
was 9, a very high-grade tumor. The bone scan and CT scan were
both normal.

Dan consulted two urologists, and both recommended he undergo a radical prostatectomy. He had one important question:
Has my cancer spread? Dan was frustrated that neither doctor
could answer that question.

I understood both Dan's frustration and the difficulty of the
urologists to provide a definitive answer. But Dan was used to
precise answers. The urologists were concerned that whatever
treatment he received would probably not be curative, but they
wanted to offer him the most definitive therapy. The treatment
that they were most comfortable recommending was what they
thought had the highest chance of cure: a radical prostatectomy.

After reviewing the clinical and pathological information and
examining Dan, I felt there was no overt evidence of spread indicated by the CT or bone scan; his PSA, when repeated, was 37.0
ng/ml. The Gleason score 9 cancer was present in three core
samples from the right side of his prostate. Dan's cancer was
easily palpable and in fact may have extended beyond the pros-

tate itself. I ordered an MRI, and it suggested extracapsular extension on the right side. This strongly indicated that a radical prostatectomy would not be curative.

I told Dan I was very concerned about his cancer. It was aggressive; it had probably advanced beyond the confines of the prostate; and there was a high degree of probability it had metastasized, although we could not yet see it. I added that I did not feel that surgery would be curative. He asked me how sure I was. I couldn't be certain, but I thought there was a greater than 90 percent chance that the surgery would not cure him.

I gave him several options to consider, one being the examination of the lymph nodes either laparoscopically or with an open surgical approach. If the lymph nodes had cancer, we could be absolutely sure of metastatic spread. I also explained that even if the lymph nodes did not reveal cancer, the cancer had a high probability of recurring in the future, so, in his case, I didn't feel compelled to recommend this examination.

His second option was surgery, which I had problems with because I feel that a radical prostatectomy (or any cancer surgery) is a procedure to remove the whole cancer, which, in Dan's case, I felt was very unlikely to occur.

A third option was radiation. This might control the cancer in the prostate, but still did not address the big issue, which was metastasis that had probably already occurred, but was not yet seen.

Lastly, the most aggressive approach was combining hormone therapy with radiation or surgery. Dan asked if I felt this was better than using radiation or surgery alone, and using hormone therapy later if he needed it. I told him that the control of the tumor in the prostate might be better, but no one knew if this approach would increase his possibility of cure.

Dan recognized the aggressiveness of his tumor and the uncertain benefits of treatment. He did not want to opt for a treatment that might well impact his quality of life for little gain. After much deliberation, he concluded: "I want to go ahead with radiation therapy then. If I need hormone treatment later, I'll do it. I don't want to start it now."

He underwent a total of thirty-seven radiation treatment sessions. During this therapy, Dan experienced limited urinary urgency and fatigue, common temporary side effects of radiation therapy.

Dan tried to maintain his professional schedule during therapy, but the fatigue caught up with him, and he decided to take off a month to recuperate. After a few weeks, he felt his normal energy level returning.

Over the next year, his energy increased to the point that he was able to conduct his normal business day, which often involved putting in up to sixteen hours making his sales rounds across New England.

Dan suffered no sexual dysfunction as a result of radiation therapy. His PSA level steadily declined following radiation therapy from a pretreatment high of 37.0 ng/ml.

When I saw Dan a year and two months after treatment, his PSA was 2.0 ng/ml and his prostate felt normal. He was heartened that his PSA level had dropped this low, but still had important questions.

First he wanted to know how low his PSA would go, referring to its downward trend. Because his PSA was so high to begin with, I explained, it could take a considerable period until it dropped to its lowest point.

"How low is good enough?" Dan persisted.

I hesitated to name an arbitrary figure because I did not want to raise unreasonable expectations, but I intended to be honest and straightforward. Dan needed information so that he could plan his future, but I knew that he'd had a rough couple of months adjusting to the gravity of his initial diagnosis and the prognosis.

As long as his PSA level was decreasing, I explained, I was pleased. This indicated that the radiation had been effective. And I hoped his PSA would continue dropping. But I needed to remind him that his cancer presented a tough problem, that clearly the main determinant of the future was the inherent aggressiveness of the tumor. I repeated that it looked as if the radiation was doing its job. If the cancer came back, I added, we would deal with it, but it was important for him to move on with his life.

Dan knew metastatic prostate cancer could not be cured. And he also recognized that the high grade of the cancer at the time of diagnosis was not a promising factor. But he also knew he had made the correct choice for himself. Following radiation therapy for prostate cancer, there is often a long period of ambiguity that both the patient and his physician must endure.

I told Dan I would periodically reevaluate him. When he left my office, he seemed to have regained an energetic bounce in his walk. He was facing a still uncertain future with courage.

Since then, Dan's cancer has remained in remission. His PSA has leveled off below 2.0 ng/ml. When it begins to rise, we will know his remission has ended.

Alternative Treatments

Any form of treatment for early, nonmetastatic prostate cancer should have the goal of either curing you or at least delaying the recurrence of the cancer long enough that it will not impact the quality of your life or your life expectancy. Keep this in mind as we discuss these alternative treatments.

Hormonal Therapy Alone

Hormonal therapy is another option in treating early, localized prostate cancer. We will spend considerable time later discussing hormonal therapy for metastatic prostate cancer. But now I'll briefly explain how hormonal therapy can also be used in men with early prostate cancer.

First let's look at the basic principle of the treatment. Prostate cancer cells require male hormones, androgens — most notably testosterone — in order to grow. When you remove or greatly reduce this male hormone from your system, most prostate cancer cells will die. Since most of your testosterone is produced in your testicles, their surgical removal (orchiectomy) would certainly abolish your primary source of androgen production. But this procedure is rarely used to lower hormone levels in cases of early, nonmetastatic prostate cancer.

Instead, some doctors use medications to disrupt the body's complex internal chemical messengers on which testosterone production depends. Monthly injections of this medication, called the luteinizing hormone-releasing hormone (LH-RH) analog (brand names Lupron and Zoladex), suppress your pituitary gland, which in turn suppresses testosterone production by your testes. This dramatically reduces your serum androgen levels (*see figure 20*).

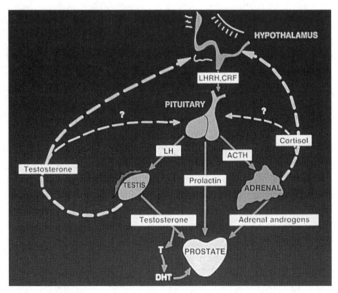

20. The LH-RH androgen system reveals the pathways among the brain, pituitary gland, testicles, and adrenal glands.
(Courtesy, Schering Corporation)

LH-RH therapy, however, has a major side effect: loss of your libido, or sex drive. Remember, your sex drive depends on the level of male hormones circulating in your blood. If the testicular production of those hormones is shut down, your sex drive drops.

Another group of oral medications, called antiandrogens, which includes flutamide (Eulexin) and bicalutamide (Casodex), does not stop testosterone production. However, these drugs do interfere with the hormone's effect on prostate cells. They will give you a similar but probably less powerful effect as either LH-RH analogs or orchiectomy, but with fewer side effects. Frequently flutamide or bicalutamide are used in conjunction with LH-RH analogs or orchiectomy (see Chapter 10).

The principle behind both these treatments is the same: your prostate epithelial cells — benign and cancerous — will be starved of the "food" they need to survive. If they all die, you're free of cancer. But hormonal deprivation does not kill all prostate cancer cells. With rare exceptions, some small amount of cancerous tissue remains in the body. Therefore, hormonal therapy cannot be considered a cure for early prostate cancer in the way radical prostatectomy or radiation therapy are. But hormonal deprivation treatment may provide a great enough reduction of the total number of cancer cells to be an appropriate therapy for some patients. In fact, as we'll see in our detailed discussion of advanced disease, hormonal therapy frequently produces this type of remission in patients with metastatic prostate cancer.

Hormonal therapy for early prostate cancer has been used in conjunction with watchful waiting — typically in older men — if and when they begin to experience symptoms. This combination of postdiagnosis observation, which often lasts for a number of years, followed by hormonal therapy, is used more frequently abroad than in the United States. This is because American medicine tends to treat prostate cancer more aggressively.

Hormonal therapy as a primary treatment strategy might be appropriate for you if you're an older man whose prostate is enlarged due to cancer and is causing symptoms but shows no evidence of metastasis (negative bone and CT scans). In this case you probably wouldn't be a reasonable candidate for initial radiation therapy or surgery because, for older men, "cure" might not be a lifesaving necessity and might not be as important as quality of life. Hormonal therapy might provide a sufficient enough remission and help relieve symptoms of the enlarged malignant prostate.

Combined Hormone Therapy

Hormonal therapy can be used in conjunction with surgery or radiation. As we noted, when used prior to surgery or radiation, your doctor might call it "neoadjuvant" or "downstaging" hormonal therapy. The benefit of this combined treatment is still under evaluation, but this approach has several possible advantages. One advantage of hormonal therapy is that it may reduce the size of your prostate and the tumor prior to surgery, making surgery less complicated and decreasing the chances that the tumor has broken through the prostate capsule or that the surgeon will leave behind cancerous tissue (positive margins).

Hormonal therapy might be used before or during radiation. The mechanism of cell death caused by hormonal therapy is different from that of radiation therapy. Therefore, combining these two treatments may increase the likelihood of killing all the cancer cells. Research studies suggest that the use of these two approaches together is more effective than radiation alone in fighting larger, more aggressive prostate cancer. The ability of this combined therapy to increase the chance of cure is unproven, however.

I offer the combined approach to very select patients — those men who are not likely to be cured with either surgery or radiation alone but who seek the most aggressive treatment. I use it also in men favoring radiation in whom the tumors are larger or more aggressive. I remind my patients that this approach is still unproven and that hormonal therapy has unpleasant side effects, including loss of sex drive, breast tenderness, and hot flashes.

Consider these factors when deciding whether combined hormonal therapy fits your needs:

- For stage C patients, hormone therapy prior to radiation would be appropriate.
- For stage A or B patients with higher PSA levels (greater than 15 ng/ml) or higher-grade levels (Gleason 8 through 10), surgery or radiation can be combined with hormone therapy.

In this scenario, you would receive hormonal therapy for a minimum of three months until the maximum effect is achieved (measured by your PSA level, evaluation of your prostate by DRE, and possibly MRI), after which you would undergo surgery or radiation.

Cryosurgery

In recent years cryosurgery, which entails freezing the prostate, has become an increasingly popular treatment option for patients with early prostate cancer. Cryosurgery has also been used for other cancers (liver tumors) with some success. In this treatment, probes containing supercold liquid nitrogen are inserted directly into the tumor. The principle of cryosurgery is that extreme cold freezes and kills cancer cells, which then will not regenerate.

If you opt for cryosurgery, a probe is inserted through the rectum in a manner similar to that of a biopsy. This treatment is a one- or two-day procedure — no doubt one reason that cryosurgery has become a popular option for treatment of localized early prostate cancer. Although this is a relatively easy treatment option and allows for other subsequent treatments if necessary, impotence is common and urinary incontinence may occur.

Are you a good candidate for cryosurgery? It's a relatively easy treatment, but side effects that occur with surgery also commonly occur with cryosurgery.

Research has not yet provided solid data to prove the long-term effectiveness of cryosurgery. Some studies show a significant decrease in PSA as well as negative biopsies following cryosurgery, which are certainly promising signs. More data is needed from larger numbers of patients with longer follow-up periods to form a reasonable opinion about the effectiveness of this therapy.

Keep these points in mind:

- Cryosurgery cannot freeze the entire prostate gland, and that is necessary in order to completely eradicate the cancer. Freezing the entire gland would damage the urethra (and adjacent sphincter), causing severe incontinence. Freezing the entire posterior part of the gland would injure the rectum, causing bowel incontinence.
- In sparing the prostate tissue adjacent to the urethra and rectum, regions of the prostate may be left untreated, and these regions may contain cancer cells.

Treatment Options — The Problem with Comparisons

Many of the treatment options for early prostate cancer may be effective, but they are difficult to compare to each other. It's reasonable for you to ask why you have so many choices and why there's so much controversy surrounding them.

Physicians who perform a certain type of therapy obviously believe in what they do. They have worked long and hard to become skilled in a demanding specialty like urology or radiation oncology. So, if you consult a urologist, he or she will probably recommend a radical prostatectomy. Radiation oncologists will favor radiation therapy. Specialists in implant treatments will suggest that type of therapy. Doctors who practice cryosurgery will offer this option.

American physicians will rarely recommend that a patient avoid therapy and opt for watchful waiting, because most patients are extremely anxious following a diagnosis of prostate cancer. Even if you're in the small group of men for whom watchful waiting may be a reasonable option, the possibility of pain and suffering (morbidity) or death occurring if you are not treated — especially considering your access to possibly curative treatments such as surgery or radiation therapy — make watchful waiting difficult to recommend. It is also more difficult for your doctor to follow your progress if you're undergoing watchful waiting than it is if you've received treatment.

Given all of this, there is considerable debate among physicians as to the optimal form of treatment. In medicine, physicians and scientists generally reach a conclusion on the best available treatment for a disease based on randomized, prospective research studies.

Doctors would benefit from data from studies in which men with prostate cancer were randomly assigned to one form of therapy or another, such as radiation or surgery. Combination therapies could be analyzed in this form of research as well. Over a course of years, this data could provide clear evidence of the comparative benefits of different forms of treatment. With some other types of cancer, such studies have established a hierarchy of recommended treatments.[1]

Because we do not yet have this data for prostate cancer, we are left with retrospective analyses of experience from a series of single institutions, which are inevitably tinged with bias. For example, one study's subjects might be younger and healthier than the typical patient. The net result is that medicine cannot say that one form of therapy had been scientifically proven to be clearly better for *you* than another.

The value of treatments must always be compared to surgery. The radical prostatectomy is the most definitive treatment for patients with early, organ-confined prostate cancer. I must stress, however, that surgery is a curative treatment only if all of your cancer is removed. And this occurs *only* in cases of organ-confined prostate cancer. If surgery does remove all your cancer, the probability of your long-term survival is very high, as high as 80 or 90 percent.

However, you may be among the men with apparent organ-confined prostate cancer who will have a recurrence of the disease after surgery. Though the pathologist may see no evidence of positive margins, seminal vesicle involvement, or lymph node involvement when he or she looks at the surgical specimen, your cancer may have already spread through the blood vessels prior to surgery and will eventually form distant metastases. We see such metastasis in about 10 to 20 percent of cases following surgery for what was thought to be organ-confined prostate cancer.

So, given an 80 to 90 percent cure rate for radical prostatectomy in cases of organ-confined prostate cancer, you should compare all other forms of treatment to surgery. It is indeed the gold standard.

You should know that the results of surgery are biased because postprostatectomy patients are analyzed on the basis of the pathological stage of their cancer. After surgery, a pathologist can establish with certainty the stage of the removed prostate and accurately say that Mr. Smith's cancer was organ confined, while Mr. Brown's had already spread to the margins and seminal vesicles. So the chances of curing organ-confined prostate cancer can be much better estimated after surgery than after other forms of surgery that do not remove the gland for later pathological examination.

Radiation therapy does not call for the removal of the prostate gland; nor do alternative treatments such as cryosurgery. Some of the men who receive these treatments will not have localized prostate cancer but rather a more advanced disease to begin with. However, researchers place these patients in the localized prostate cancer category, making direct comparisons difficult.

Preferred Forms of Treatment: My Recommendations

I would recommend that you have a radical prostatectomy if you have a long life expectancy and appear to have a high likelihood of cure following a complete pretreatment diagnostic workup. This includes the PSA, DRE, biopsy, pathological staging, bone scan, and perhaps MRI. I recommend surgery only to those who fully understand and accept the side effects of this treatment. Remember, surgery is a good but not perfect form of treatment: the side effects are significant.

I might recommend radiation to you as a reasonable form of therapy if I felt your likelihood of cure was high and you expressed that you did not want to endure the side effects of surgery. Most men fear the side effect of urinary incontinence more than sexual impotence. I tell them that surgery might be a more effective treatment than external-beam radiation, but that the potential benefits gained with surgery are a tradeoff for its side effects. Radioactive seeds or implants may be ideal for this group of patients.

I also recommend radiation if your diagnostic workup suggests that you are unlikely to be cured by surgery. In this case you might show no clear evidence of metastatic disease but you have a high likelihood of "occult" or hidden metastasis because your PSA is above 15.0 ng/ml, you have a high-grade cancer with a Gleason score of perhaps 8, 9, or 10, or you have a stage C tumor. Generally I do not feel cases such as these can be cured by surgery. So rather than have you undergo surgery, which has inevitable side effects, and in this case, a low likelihood of cure, I would recommend radiation therapy as more appropriate for you. For such patients I frequently recommend external-beam radiation in conjunction with hormonal therapy. You might not be cured of prostate cancer under these conditions, but there is a good chance that this combined therapy would work for a long length of time.

If your physicians believe from your diagnostic workup that you have a low probability of being cured by surgery, I would not recommend it. I'd also avoid surgery if you're elderly or have other health problems that might make surgery life threatening.

If your individual situation doesn't fit any of these general categories, try to obtain as much information about your condition as possible, and once again, ask about the likelihood of your being cured and get an estimate of your life expectancy, as best your physicians can determine.

Watchful Waiting: Theoretical Considerations

One possible scenario for prostate cancer is that a microscopic malignancy — which poses you no immediate threat — will grow to a big, aggressive cancer that could shorten your life. In other words, some oncologists think a tiny "indolent" cancer, if left untreated, will one day become big and dangerous — if you live long enough. But this progression from harmless to life threatening is not well understood in terms of how long it takes and whether modification in our lifestyle might change this process. I think it is also likely that some people start off with a small, aggressive cancer, which is not likely to be very modifiable with lifestyle changes. So we can say prostate cancer has a heterogeneous — uncertain — natural history.

There is a great difference in the tumor growth rate among different men. Think of a tumor growing from a microscopic single cell to a much bigger mass. If its growth rate is measured in the doubling times of total cells or in tumor volume, we see a wide variety in progression rates, as measured in PSA levels. Doubling occurs in only a few months in certain men but may take years in others. This suggests either that there is more than one biological route involved in the progression of prostate cancer or that some tumors acquire mutations quicker than others.

This lack of knowledge makes your treatment decision more

difficult. Do keep these three principles in mind if you're considering watchful waiting:

- In general, smaller, lower-grade tumors grow more slowly than larger tumors.
- Tumors that are larger and higher-grade at the time of diagnosis will probably grow more quickly and become more dangerous.
- Younger men have a longer future for their cancer to grow and become aggressive. There is reason to believe that, *in general,* prostate cancers that occur in younger men may be more aggressive to begin with and therefore should be treated.

Watchful Waiting: Practical Considerations

Given the diverse progression rate of prostate tumors, your cancer might be growing so slowly that you're likely to die of other causes before the tumor becomes life threatening. It would certainly be a giant step forward in the management of prostate cancer if we could identify cancers with such low metastatic potential. If your doctor could predict that your small, low-grade cancer would remain indolent and organ-confined, he could safely recommend watchful waiting.

Such an ability would be especially important, given the increased incidence of diagnosed prostate cancer. Presumably, as the screening net is cast in a broader arc, doctors will diagnose a greater proportion of these "unimportant" cancers, tumors that have a very slow growth rate and will not compromise men's life expectancy.

On one side of this issue is your realistic life expectancy at the time of screening and diagnosis. Unfortunately, we have only very crude methods of measuring how long you or anybody else will survive. These estimates can be made, but they are difficult to make in individual patients. As we increase in age, life expectancy decreases. The average life expectancy of a 25-year-old man is 50 years, while his 50-year-old father has a life expectancy of 25 years. Currently, the life expectancy of a 70-year-old man is twelve or thirteen years.

If you've been diagnosed with early prostate cancer, is your life expectancy greater or less than the projected natural history of the tumor? Certainly your other health problems enter the equation, though it isn't easy to weigh their impact. Presently, you can live for years being treated for cardiovascular disease that might have been life threatening only a decade ago.

Your life expectancy is critical in determining whether you should be treated for localized prostate cancer. A cancer that might require thirty years to become dangerous is not life threatening if your life expectancy at the time of diagnosis is twenty years.

To form your best judgment in this situation, you have to better define two elements in the equation. One is obviously your individual life expectancy. The other is determining how aggressive your cancer is — that is, how likely it is to spread.

You can immediately form one conclusion: a short life expectancy should preclude aggressive treatment. If you're a man with a severe life-threatening illness or you're in your mid- to late-70s and have recently been diagnosed with organ-confined prostate cancer and have no symptoms, you should *not* undergo aggressive therapy for your localized prostate cancer.

Unfortunately, it is difficult to assess a tumor's metastatic potential. Your doctors cannot determine precisely how aggressive your cancer is. It is possible that a slowly growing cancer might metastasize. Thus there is not a firm correlation between apparent growth rate and metastatic potential.

Research findings are not yet conclusive but strongly suggest the following points to consider:

- There is probably a relationship between tumor volume (measured in cubic centimeters) and the degree of cell differentiation; hence your tumor volume may be a useful predictor of metastatic potential.

- In general, prostate cancers with a volume of less than 1 cubic centimeter have a low metastatic potential; tumors smaller than 3.5 cubic centimeters rarely penetrate the prostate capsule and invade the seminal vesicles.
- Prostate tumors larger than 5 cubic centimeters usually contain relatively more poorly differentiated cells and are thus more metastatically aggressive.

Conversely, it is dangerous to assume that *all* small-volume tumors are destined to remain of low metastatic potential. Not all small (low-volume), low-grade tumors will definitely remain harmless for the rest of one's life. Equally, if you have an organ-confined tumor greater than 5 cubic centimeters in volume, it might not grow and metastasize rapidly.[2]

In some men, the tumor growth rate is rapid from the beginning, and this growth rate remains consistent throughout the course of their disease. Research also indicates that there are many men who have very slow-growing tumors that never acquire a rapid growth rate. Obviously there is diverse biological potential among individual prostate cancers. In some men, there may be an acceleration of tumor growth over a period of time; in others, the cancer grows slowly throughout its natural history and never metastasizes.[3]

Research studies also suggest that if you have a high-grade but apparently localized prostate cancer at the time of diagnosis, you are not a good candidate for watchful waiting if your life expectancy is greater than ten years.[4]

Before you decide for or against watchful waiting, let's look more closely at the two different strategies that can be employed in the process.

The first is basically no treatment; no close observation or regular monitoring through DREs or PSA assays occurs. You try to resume your life almost as if you have not been diagnosed with localized prostate cancer. Only when — or if — it becomes clinically apparent through symptoms of pain or urinary obstruction that the disease has progressed does your physician intervene with treatment, which is generally palliative (alleviating symptoms), not curative. You should consider this more passive approach:

- If you have no symptoms and a limited life expectancy due to advanced age, you should probably defer aggressive therapy.
- If you are younger and have another serious health problem (such as severe diabetes or cardiovascular disease).

The second strategy I call deferred treatment. Treatment might eventually become appropriate for you, but the characteristics of your cancer indicate that the cancer poses no risk. Deferred treatment involves close monitoring through regular PSA assays, DREs, and perhaps repeat biopsies of the prostate to see if the volume and/or grade of your tumor have significantly changed.

Case History: Tom Alexander

Veteran journalist Tom Alexander presented this dilemma in a very personal manner in a *Fortune* article in 1993. Alexander, who had just retired at age 62, underwent a routine physical that included a PSA assay. His PSA level was 5.9 ng/ml, which prompted further tests, including an ultrasound-guided biopsy. He received a pathological diagnosis of prostate cancer with a low-volume, Gleason score 3 + 2 tumor confined to one lobe of the gland.

Alexander researched his treatment options for several months. He encountered the full gamut of confusion — what he called the "rampant disarray" — when seeking information about the best treatment for his cancer. The assistant to one very prominent urologist returned Alexander's call late at night and announced, "You need to get into surgery right away. If you don't, the chances are about 100 percent that your cancer will escape the prostate in the next one to two years." Clearly this urological practice was sold on the radical prostatectomy. Radiation therapists also swore by their treatment, stressing that it minimized the risk of impotence.

Alexander then consulted with the late Willet E. Whitmore, one of the senior figures in contemporary urology. Whitmore reminded Alexander, "Growing old is invariably fatal, while prostate cancer is only sometimes so." But Whitmore also leaned heavily toward a radical prostatectomy in Alexander's particular case, in which it seemed the tumor was most probably still organ confined.

Alexander continued to seek other opinions. Along the way, he encountered men in patient support groups who complained bitterly that they had been rushed into surgery without a full understanding of possible side effects. One man who had undergone a radical prostatectomy only to later be diagnosed with metastatic disease was both impotent and incontinent. He lamented, "I wish I had taken more time."

Tom Alexander was more concerned about the side effects than a malignant tumor in his prostate. Eventually he consulted Dr. Jonathan Jarow at the Bowman Gray Hospital in Winston-Salem, North Carolina, and together they devised an appropriate watchful waiting strategy that involved careful monitoring. After a diagnostic workup that excluded the presence of metastatic disease, they settled on a contingency plan. Alexander would undergo periodic PSA assays and DREs. If the PSA rose toward 10.0 ng/ml or the tumor obviously increased in volume, he would reconsider treatment.

Whether such a course is appropriate if you have a similar diagnosis is up to you and your physician. The best manner of following people like this has not been determined. Using a PSA value of 10.0 provides a practical benchmark, but one must realize that this is arbitrary.

Again, an important principle applies: treatment is an investment in the future. In this deferred treatment approach, you and your physician often decide in advance on a contingency plan to reconsider treatment if your cancer seems to be progressing beyond the incidental local stage. Your treatment is therefore deferred until a time when your need for therapy may be clearer. You might choose a certain PSA value or a rate of change of PSA (PSA velocity), or a change in your DRE, or a pathological finding from the biopsies as your decision point.

This strategy is also somewhat arbitrary; it is not based on any research that clearly defines the appropriate time to start your active treatment. Studies comparing watchful waiting with surgery or radiation therapy in the United States will not produce results for several more years.

You might consider the deferred treatment strategy of watchful waiting if a thorough diagnostic workup indicates you have a low-volume, low-grade cancer, for example, or if only one of your multiple biopsy cores shows cancer and the cancer is present in only a small part of the core and there is no Gleason 7 or higher. I would still be hesitant to recommend this approach, however, if you have a long life expectancy.

Researchers stress that many prostate cancers detected through PSA screening in men older than 70 are not clinically significant. But many men over the age of 70 feel pressure to choose among competing treatment options. A recent study published in the *Journal of the American Medical Association* summarizes the issue: "One concern about screening for prostate cancer is that it might detect low-grade, low-volume cancers that may progress so slowly that they do not pose an immediate threat to the patient."

A major study of prostate cancer, the Patient Outcomes Research Team (PORT), strongly favors watchful waiting for the older patient: "One finding is very clear: men aged 75 years or older are not likely to benefit from either radiation therapy or radical prostatectomy when compared with watchful waiting."

When I consult men in this age group, I often recommend watchful waiting. Some find it psychologically unacceptable to leave their cancer untreated, and they might choose radiation therapy or hormonal therapy treatment. The choice of watchful waiting over surgery or radiation therapy is much more troubling for younger patients. Certainly, if you have a life expectancy of greater than ten years and you choose watchful waiting, the deferred treatment approach involving active monitoring of the disease is reasonable. Many doctors recommend follow-up testing involving DREs and PSAs every four to twelve months, with annual biopsies. If your PSA steadily rises over time or changes at a brisk pace, or if your DRE reveals a newly palpable mass, it is reasonable to assume your tumor is advancing. In this case you may decide on surgery or radiation therapy.

There is a risk, unfortunately, that therapy might not cure you at that point. This is because, as we've discussed, metastatic spread is an unpredictable process. What seemed like an obviously low-grade, low-volume tumor confined to a single lobe of your gland might actually have been part of a more diffuse malignancy with more aggressive portions of the cancer in areas that were not biopsied.

Therefore, we are again faced with a complex issue about which you and your physician should communicate as honestly as possible. If you opt for deferred therapy when diagnosed with apparently localized prostate cancer, you should be aware that you may be missing the opportunity for a cure. The chances of missing an opportunity for cure decrease as we get older and are less likely for men with slow-growing cancers.

If you are a vigorous, otherwise healthy man in your fifties who has just been diagnosed with a low-grade, low-volume prostate tumor, the issue becomes even more difficult. Perhaps as part of the very human psychological reflex we call denial, you will opt for a few more "good years" before you undergo the side effects of treatment. And you might seek comfort in the hope that the low Gleason score of your tumor and its apparent low volume *guarantee* that this cancer will remain indolent for several years. Unfortunately, there are not many guarantees in this business.

Perhaps you definitely want to be cured but you don't want to face the side effects of treatment immediately. This is understandable. I often consult men who are in this emotional bind, distraught because the impact of treatment will be appreciated many years later, while the side effects must be endured immediately. If you have this dilemma, try to bear in mind that side effects can be alleviated, but metastatic prostate cancer cannot be cured.

The key factor in choosing among your treatment options (watchful waiting, surgery, or radiation therapy) is to form the best estimate about your prostate tumor's metastatic potential. For example, if we could have determined with some degree of certainty that Bill J.'s seemingly localized, low-volume, low-grade cancer would not spread beyond the prostate gland before the end of his normal life expectancy, then recommending against radical prostatectomy, radiation therapy, or any form of treatment in favor of watchful waiting would have been relatively straightforward. But estimating the metastatic potential of prostate cancer is not easy.

When considering watchful waiting, try to obtain an estimate of your tumor's metastatic potential based on known factors. I hope that in the future we will rely more heavily on the genetic constitution of the malignancy to give us more information.

Case History: Deferred Therapy

Larry M. is a self-employed commercial fisherman, age 70. He is in reasonably good general health, although he was able to break a lifelong addiction to cigarettes only recently. Over the course of the past fifteen years, he noted that his urinary stream had slowed and he'd been getting up to urinate twice each night.

During a physical examination Larry's physician conducted a DRE, which revealed an enlarged prostate of symmetrical shape and smooth texture. This was indicative of relatively moderate

BPH. With Larry's permission, the physician drew a PSA assay, which produced a level of 6.0 ng/ml. Although high, the PSA level was consistent with his age and BPH. The physician had the test repeated six months later. Now the PSA level had risen to 6.5 ng/ml. But the next DRE and an ultrasonic imaging did not indicate the prostate had grown significantly larger through BPH. The doctor recommended prostate biopsies.

The urologist conducting the biopsy took eight core samples. The pathological examination of these samples detected cancer in one core taken from the center of the right posterior lobe. The grade of this cancer was low, Gleason 2 + 2, and the estimated volume of the tumor was very small, based on the fact that only 5 percent of the single-core biopsy that was positive actually contained cancer.

Larry, who is a widower, came to see me with his oldest son, with whom he works. After a staging evaluation, including a bone scan that was negative, I explained that the tumor appeared to be very small and was low-grade. Larry's treatment options included radiation therapy, radical prostatectomy, and watchful waiting.

Larry asked if he should make an immediate decision, considering the fact that his cancer didn't appear to be dangerous. I could see that he was worried about the side effects of treatment — the threat of incontinence and sexual dysfunction.

"I don't think you need to make a decision immediately. The tumor doesn't appear to be dangerous at this point," I said. "But I can't predict reliably how the cancer will behave over the long term."

Larry and his son understood the situation. Together we worked out a strategy for watchful waiting. Larry would repeat DREs and PSA assays every six months. If the tumor became palpable in the DRE or his PSA rose above 8.0 ng/ml, he would undergo radiation therapy. We also planned on repeating the biopsies in a year. In the meantime, he began a course of the medication Hytrin to alleviate his symptoms of BPH.

I last saw Larry a few months ago, and he was doing well. His symptoms have improved. His PSA is 6.2 ng/ml; his DREs reveal that his prostate is still smooth and symmetrical.

At this time we will continue to observe Larry's cancer, repeating the biopsies when he returns, and defer treatment.

9

Life after Treatment

Posttreatment Evaluations

If you are treated for early prostate cancer by radical prostatectomy, radiation therapy, or other forms of therapy, you will undergo posttreatment evaluations to make sure that treatment has been effective and to verify that recovery is taking place. In the case of surgery, your first evaluation will take place several weeks following discharge from the hospital. After radiation therapy, your first follow-up evaluation occurs within a few months.

As with pretreatment diagnosis, the DRE and the PSA blood test are the principal methods used to assess the effectiveness of your therapy. What your physician discovers from these two techniques will differ depending on the type of treatment you had. Generally, these examinations will be repeated every three months for a year or so following either radical prostatectomy or radiation therapy, and usually less frequently thereafter. The hope, of course, is that no signs of your cancer return. Although these visits can be worrisome, look at them as potentially reassuring.

Postsurgery — Was I Cured?

Your physician will probably give you a physical exam, including a DRE, following radical prostatectomy, even though you no longer have a prostate gland to palpate. Instead, your doctor is feeling the postsurgical prostatic fossa — the area in which your prostate was situated. The purpose of this DRE is to determine if there is any palpable recurrent growth of tumor in this area, which is not likely. Your physician will note any changes in comparison with subsequent DREs. If your doctor detects suspicious-feeling tissue (especially hard nodules) during these DREs, he or she might be concerned that residual cancer remains in your pelvis. If this occurs, a biopsy might be performed.

Postsurgery: The PSA

Your PSA test after radical prostatectomy is a much more telling test than the DRE. Following surgery to remove the entire prostate gland, the serum level of your PSA assay should be below detectable levels, which may vary from one laboratory to another. This can be below 0.3 ng/ml, below 0.1 ng/ml, or simply an indication that no PSA was detected in your blood.

The serum level drops to virtually zero following a successful radical prostatectomy because there are no longer any prostate epithelial cells present in the body to produce the PSA protein; if the surgery was successful, all such tissue should have been removed.

If the PSA is detectable in your blood following surgery, however, this almost always means that malignant prostate cells producing PSA have remained in your body (persistent residual prostate cancer). But this residual cancer might not yet have spread to distant sites beyond your pelvis.

Circumstances of detectable PSA following surgery can vary. You may have persistently detectable PSA beginning with your first assay following the prostatectomy. Or you may have an undetectable level soon after surgery, but it begins to rise in subsequent PSA assays (months or years later). The actual level of detectable PSA in your blood is less important than the existence of a rising trend. But remember that fluctuations may be due to variations from one lab to the next.

A rising PSA level, whether it be 0.0 to 0.1 to 0.2 to 0.3 ng/ml or 0.0 to 1 to 5 to 10 ng/ml, suggests that you have persistent cancer. If this is the case, your physician may order more tests, including a bone scan, to help determine if the residual prostate cancer has visibly spread to other parts of your body. Under most circumstances when persistent cancer is detected this way, the bone scan shows no cancer.

In some patients, persistent postsurgical cancer will be strictly limited to the region of the prostate. This means the cancer has not yet metastasized. But prostate cancer specialists find that in most men with detectable and rising PSA following surgery, the cancer has spread beyond the region of the prostate even if the bone scan reveals no cancer. If you have detectable PSA after surgery, your doctor may order an MRI scan to look for a local recurrence. A bone scan is useful in determining whether the cancer in your body has metastasized to bone. However, if you have only a few cancer cells producing detectable PSA after surgery, they won't yet appear as obvious tumor sites on the scan.

If your pathology report indicates cancer is present at a surgical margin (positive margins), there is probably residual cancer locally, particularly if your PSA is elevated. The larger question is whether malignant cells are limited to this site or whether the cancer has metastasized. Further, high-grade cancers (Gleason 8 through 10) and those that have invaded the seminal vesicles as revealed in the postsurgical pathological report are more likely to metastasize.

In the case of a rising PSA after surgery, two other methods — biopsies and radionuclide scanning — can be used to help distinguish between a recurrence just near the prostate and the existence of metastatic disease. Your doctor may want to perform a biopsy of the anastomosis site (where the bladder links to the urethra). If the biopsy is positive, that is pretty good confirmation of local recurrence, but does not rule out that some cancer cells have metastasized.

Radionuclide scanning, a recent innovation, involves tagging antibodies to proteins on the surface of prostate cancer cells with radioactive tracers much like in the bone scan. These proteins will attach only if prostate cells are still present in your body. This test is still in evolution, but you may ask your physician about it if your PSA is elevated after surgery.

It is hoped that your PSA will remain undetectable the rest of your life. There is no better sign than this. However, if your PSA becomes detectable, the length of time after treatment that PSA is first detected and its speed of increase will tell you and your doctors something about the growth rate of the residual tumor. If your PSA remains undetectable for two years and then begins to climb, taking two more years to double, you have a slower tumor growth rate than someone in whom the PSA is detectable three months after surgery and is doubling every month.

If bone metastases fail to appear on one scan despite a rising PSA trend, you and your physician might consider follow-up radiation therapy after surgery. As mentioned, this is particularly true if your postprostatectomy pathology report revealed close or positive surgical margins. In this case it is possible that the relatively small amount of residual malignant tissue is localized in your pelvis, adjacent to the former position of the prostate, and thus can be effectively reached by external-beam radiation.

You also may benefit from hormonal therapy, but there are currently no data to prove that such therapy provides a cure. However, there is a growing tendency to use hormonal therapy earlier than later.

Important points to remember following treatment:

- If you have a detectable or rising PSA following a radical prostatectomy, discuss the situation thoroughly with your physician. Request a detailed explanation of the postsurgical pathological findings. You should fully understand whether the cancer appeared to be organ confined or whether it extended beyond the prostate, through the capsule, to the margins, or into the seminal vesicles.
- Don't be embarrassed to request simplified anatomical dia-

grams or models if you do not understand the structures of your body the physician is discussing. You and your family have a right to be as well informed as possible about your posttreatment prognosis.

- All this information is important in judging whether a persistent cancer indicated by the detectable PSA has remained localized in your pelvis or has metastasized. Your physician should share with you his or her best judgment on this important question. And you, as an informed patient, should be able to participate in the decisions on appropriate follow-up treatment.

As you undergo posttreatment evaluations, bear in mind that the PSA assay has changed the way we manage patients after treatment, either radical prostatectomy or radiation therapy. Just as the widespread use of the PSA test has altered our concept of prostate cancer detection and assigning appropriate therapy, the PSA test has also become the most important method of determining whether your treatment has been effective. If radical prostatectomy has cured you, your PSA level should remain undetectable the rest of your life.

To put this into perspective, before the advent of the PSA test, patients undergoing treatment would have been assumed cured under most circumstances. For example, a man who'd had a radical prostatectomy and did not have any evidence of metastatic disease would have been considered free of the disease because the only means of learning that the treatment had failed was by scans, not the PSA test.

A significant number of patients are confronted with convincing evidence — detectable or rising levels of PSA — that they have persistent cancer following surgery. Not surprisingly, this often creates extreme anxiety; these men have undergone considerable discomfort and anguish and have accepted the probability of the side effects of treatment, only to find that the reassurance of a complete cure has eluded them.

Adjuvant Hormone Therapy

One concept that has yet to be fully explored for prostate cancer is the use of hormone therapy for a period after receiving local treatment. The hope is that this treatment will decrease the likelihood of the cancer's recurrence. Adjuvant hormone therapy has been shown to be effective for breast cancer in women: Tamoxifen, a hormonal drug, will decrease the likelihood of recurrence and increase survival slightly in women with breast cancer after they have received surgery or radiation. We don't yet know the effect of hormonal drugs on men with prostate cancer who have just undergone surgery or radiation. At the moment, I don't recommend it routinely.

Follow-up Therapy

If you learn that you have a residual tumor, don't give in to despair. The fact that you might have a detectable PSA level after radical prostatectomy does not necessarily mean that you are incurable. Your residual cancer might be localized to your pelvis.

On the positive side, the use of the posttreatment PSA has led physicians to detect persistent cancer earlier and to aggressively treat it, hoping to eradicate the persistent cancer that is producing the PSA. Such is the rationale behind the use of radiation and early hormonal therapy in postprostatectomy patients with detectable PSA.

If the margins of your surgically removed prostate showed cancer and the serum level of your PSA is detectable, radiation therapy to the pelvis will probably decrease your PSA level. You might then have an undetectable PSA level for years after follow-up radiation therapy. Unfortunately, the chances are greater than 50 percent that radiation therapy will not completely eradicate the cancer under such circumstances.

Nevertheless, if the surgical margins (other than the urethral margin) following radical prostatectomy are positive — with or without detectable PSA — I would recommend radiation therapy for you. If pathological examination reveals the cancer has penetrated the capsule (with no positive margins), in the absence of detectable postsurgery PSA, I would recommend a more conservative course to you. If you had a detectable postoperative PSA level, I'd recommend only radiation. If you have only penetration of the capsule, this does not necessarily mean your cancer will return.

If a tumor has invaded the seminal vesicles, the cancer has likely spread to other parts of the body. The reasons for this are unclear, but experience has lead us to this conclusion. Therefore, if the postsurgery pathological examination detects malignancy in one or both of your seminal vesicles, I do not usually recommend postoperative radiation therapy. The question for you now is whether or not to begin adjuvant hormonal therapy, the benefits of which are still uncertain.

When radiation is used after surgery, the course is similar to that given if your prostate were in place: the radiation oncology team plans the radiation based on where the organ had been. In general, the dose of radiation is slightly less and the field slightly smaller than the course you would have received prior to the removal of your prostate. Radiation therapy after surgery may worsen existing urinary incontinence and impotence and may cause a change in bowel habits.

Radiation Therapy: The Posttreatment Physical Exam

Changes usually occur slowly after radiation, and even with complete eradication of the tumor in your prostate, the gland may still feel abnormal. It can take many months, if not longer, for the prostate gland returns to normal. Therefore, the DRE is not a good diagnostic technique immediately after radiation therapy, and the results can be difficult to interpret.

The PSA

After radiation therapy, either external-beam or implant, your PSA level should steadily decrease. It would be very unusual, however, to see a quick posttreatment drop in your PSA to undetectable levels, as is often the case following radical prostatectomy.

To understand why an elevated PSA level often persists after treatment, you must understand the biological effect of radiation on prostate cells, both malignant and normal. Theoretically, radiation will be more destructive to malignant than to normal tissue because cancer cells are more likely to be damaged by, or are less capable of repairing the damage caused by radiation, than their benign counterparts. However, radiation does not immediately kill all the vulnerable malignant cells. Some may survive for a period of months following treatment.

Your normal prostate cells, unlike cancerous cells, might be in a dormant state and relatively insensitive to radiation. So you can almost always expect a certain number of normal prostate cells to survive radiation therapy, with cancerous cells dying progressively over time.

With some of your prostate epithelial tissue surviving radiation therapy, it is unusual for your PSA level to drop to virtually zero. Your immediate postradiation PSA values, however, should be lower than pretreatment levels. And your subsequent PSA assays should show a downward trend. It may take months for your PSA level to drop to its lowest value.

The lower your PSA level falls after radiation therapy, the more likely it is that your cancer has been eradicated. We don't know the optimal level of decrease, but a PSA level below 1.0 ng/ml is desirable. However, there certainly are men who have levels higher than 1.0 ng/ml after radiation therapy who never relapse.

A rising trend in PSA level after radiation therapy indicates persistent disease, as it does after radical prostatectomy. If your PSA begins to rise after radiation therapy, your physician should try to determine if you have persistent disease only in your prostate or elsewhere in your body. This evaluation may be inconclusive, however. If it appears that the tumor has persisted only in the prostate, you might consider the most aggressive approach: a salvage prostatectomy. Unfortunately, this surgery cures few patients and has major side effects. Impotence is typical; permanent incontinence is common. Rectal injury (requiring a colostomy) is unusual, but there is a risk that it will occur. If your doctors recommended radiation therapy originally, you probably were not an appropriate candidate for radical prostatectomy to begin with. I rarely recommend the postradiation salvage prostatectomy.

Other forms of local therapy, such as cryosurgery, may be considered. Cryosurgery's effectiveness under these circumstances is uncertain; in addition, urinary incontinence and impotence are common.

If you've undergone either radical prostatectomy or radiation therapy, routine follow-up bone scans are not necessary unless your PSA has shown a rising trend or unless symptoms occur, such as pain that persists and is unexplained. If a follow-up bone scan shows that the cancer has spread to your bone, further treatment to the prostate is not needed and you should definitely consider hormonal therapy (see Chapter 10).

Treating Side Effects from Primary Therapy: Urinary Incontinence

The bladder is a muscular pouch connected to a system of adjacent muscles that surround the prostate in the base of the pelvis. Before surgery, all these muscles act in unison to maintain urinary continence. If you undergo a radical prostatectomy, no matter how skilled your surgeon, there is bound to be some disruption in this complex system of interacting muscles; this can result in urinary incontinence of varying severity and duration.

You almost certainly will *not* suffer permanent, severe incontinence. Fewer than 5 percent of radical prostatectomy patients have lost complete control of their urine one year after treatment. And only about 20 to 30 percent of men might still need to wear a pad due to mild to moderate stress incontinence. If this problem does persist, it is important for your physician to evaluate you thoroughly. You might have an easily treated condition such as infection or blockage of the urethra from scar tissue (a urethral stricture).

If you are among the very small percentage of men who suffer severe incontinence, you have several forms of therapy available to you. The most traditional is a penile clamp, which is actually less uncomfortable than its name implies, or an external urine-collecting bag that is worn permanently.

The most effective treatment for severe incontinence is an implanted artificial sphincter. This reliable appliance requires surgery to implant, which may be a psychological obstacle if you have recently undergone another major surgical procedure. The artificial sphincter has an adjustable cuff that is fitted around the postprostatectomy urethra adjacent to the muscles of the external urethral sphincter. This cuff is connected by durable surgical-grade tubing to a small pump inserted into the scrotum and to a reservoir of biologically inert liquid that is implanted in the posterior abdominal cavity. A siphonlike action allows the urethral clamp to deflate when you activate the pump to urinate. The cufflike clamp automatically closes a short time later as liquid is returned through the tube from the reservoir.

If you're among the 20 or 30 percent of postprostatectomy men who experience the milder forms of stress incontinence, you may not be able to find a completely satisfactory solution. One easy and highly effective means of avoiding the embarrassment of stress incontinence is to get reinforced underwear. Manufacturers such as HealthDri, a subdivision of TransAqua in Charlotte, North Carolina, make underwear that accommodates different activities and different levels of incontinence. Ask your urologist to consider medications that promote contraction of smooth muscles, including Tofranil, Ditropan, or Entex.

As mentioned in Chapter 7, many men gain better control of their urine by retraining their muscles through a regimen of Kegel exercise. These exercises were developed to strengthen and coordinate your voluntary muscle groups, which in turn tone the involuntary musculature that helps maintain urinary continence through the internal urethral sphincter. Your urologist (or a designated physical therapist) can provide detailed information on the proper training course for the Kegel exercises at an appropriate time following healing from surgery. Basically, these exercises involve the voluntary muscles you use when you have to abruptly stop the urine stream, as well as the muscles behind your scrotum that you use to force out any remaining urine you feel in your penile urethra following the closing of the external urethral sphincter.

This coordination might sound complicated, but urologists and physical therapists today have clear written instructions and diagrams to help you along the training course that is most appropriate for you. Be sure to discuss Kegel exercises with your physician. Your doctor may also advocate decreasing or eliminating caffeine and alcohol and practicing complete voiding of your bladder during urination. These steps can help while you are retraining your postsurgical sphincter.

As we have noted, urinary incontinence is rare in patients treated with radiation therapy. But when it does occur, the treatment options are very similar to those discussed here.

Treating Side Effects from Primary Therapy: Sexual Dysfunction

Prostate cancer treatment, either radical prostatectomy or radiation therapy, often interferes with your erection and/or ejaculation. During erection, the nerve bundles around your prostate cause increased blood flow to fill two fibrous cylindrical tubes that lie side by side along the centerline of your upper penis. These tubes are called the corpora cavernosa or cavernous bodies. When swelled with blood the flacid penis lifts into its erect state.

The exact mechanism involved in posttreatment sexual dysfunction is not understood. But the severing of nerves that control the blood flow necessary to achieve erection, as well as disruption of the blood flow itself, is often involved. Radiation therapy can degrade this process as well.[1]

As a side effect of prostatectomy, radiation therapy, or cryosurgery, the nerves that control the blood vessels that engorge your penis during erection might be severed (in the case of surgery) or damaged (in the case of radiation therapy or cryosurgery). Treatment may have also damaged the blood vessels themselves. But you should keep in mind that these treatments do not actually damage the anatomy of your external penis. Some men stoically accept the fact that treatment may cause impotence. However, you do have options. You can achieve erection via means other than the normal nerve impulse mechanism.

The simplest treatment for impotence is the vacuum pump. This device has evolved considerably since its invention. Today, vacuum pumps that facilitate erection are reliable and easy to use. When you're ready for intercourse, you insert your flacid penis into the clear plastic cylinder of the pump and activate a hand mechanism that evacuates the air from the tube. This serves to stretch the tissue of your penis to the point where the blood vessels of the corpora cavernosa open and fill with blood. This gives you a nearly normal erection. To maintain the erection you must keep your penis engorged, so you slip a specialized rubber retaining band off the vacuum cylinder and onto the base of your penis. This band constricts the blood channel and prevents the engorged bodies from draining during intercourse. Many men find this an acceptable solution.

Another option is the use of injections of medication that serve to stimulate blood flow into the penis. You might not find the idea of injecting your penis with a needle appealing, but many men quickly adapt to this painless treatment option. The drugs, often a derivative of a naturally occurring substance called prostaglandin, are effective and easy to use. You employ a very fine syringe and needle with minimal discomfort. Other drugs you can use for self-injection are papaverine and regitine. An injection of the appropriate drug gives you a blood flow adequate for erection following sexual stimulation. Many men and their partners find this form of treatment more acceptable than vacuum devices.

If you can't be treated by the methods we have discussed, you may opt for the implanted penile prosthesis. As with the vacuum pump, these surgically implanted prostheses have evolved considerably in recent years.

The simplest prosthesis is the malleable or semi-rigid device. It consists of twin tubes of surgical-grade, pliable plastic that are implanted into your corpora cavernosa from the root to the head of your penis. Because they completely fill the two erectile bodies along the penis, the implant creates a rigid penis that is effective for intercourse. Because the tubes are malleable, you can bend your penis down along the inner thigh except during sexual activity, when you can raise your penis to the erect position. You should be heartened to know that the implant is easy to conceal.

You might want to consider a more elaborate surgically implanted prosthesis developed in recent years. Similar to the artificial urinary sphincter, this device uses a reservoir-and-pump system through which a biologically inert fluid flows. Again, paired tubes are implanted in your upper penis. But these tubes inflate with the liquid from the reservoir when the pump anchored in your scrotum is activated. After sexual intercourse, the pump deflates the implanted tubes and the liquid is returned to the reservoir, which is located in your lower abdominal cavity above the pubic bone.

Neither type of implant affects urinary function because your penile urethra is located below and separate from the corpora cavernosa.

Your ability to ejaculate semen is almost always lost after radical prostatectomy; sometimes a very small amount of fluid will be ejaculated. About one-third of radiation therapy patients can still have ejaculations following treatment. However, your ability to achieve orgasm is maintained following either prostate cancer surgery or radiation therapy. Therefore, if you can be successfully treated for the side effect of erectile dysfunction through one of the options I have outlined, you may regain much of the pleasure of sex that you experienced before treatment.

Another concern to most men is whether they will remain capable of producing sperm after treatment. Sperm is produced in the testicles, which are not affected. Although the "plumbing" is altered after surgery, sperm is still produced. Theoretically, men are capable of fertilizing an ovum after treatment using special artificial insemination techniques, but not through sexual intercourse.

Case History: John R.

Two years ago, a New England urologist referred John R. to me. John was a 58-year-old retired naval officer who now runs his own boatyard. He had undergone a physical examination and evaluation. A PSA assay obtained a level of 10.0 ng/ml. His DRE was normal, although indicative of a slightly enlarged prostate. His internist said that since John's DRE was normal and his prostate was enlarged, no further studies were warranted. John, feeling somewhat uncertain, came to the Dana-Farber Cancer Institute for a second opinion.

A repeat PSA revealed a level of 9.4 ng/ml, higher than one would find with moderate BPH in a man 58. I performed a DRE. John's prostate was only slightly enlarged. Moreover, the gland was smooth and relatively soft in texture, not indicative of an obvious tumor.

I told John that his PSA was quite high, but that I couldn't explain why without more tests. John wanted to know if he had prostate cancer. I didn't want to coddle him or unduly alarm him. I recommended that he return to his urologist for a biopsy.

John frowned when I gave him my recommendation, as he was hoping that I could tell him he didn't have cancer.

I knew that for the next few days until the biopsy results were determined, John would be very anxious. This painful uncertainty is typical. I tried to reassure him by saying that whatever the biopsy showed, the information it would provide was important, and we would have gained a better knowledge of what to do.

Two weeks after consulting me, John returned for our second discussion of his case. He brought with him a thick folder of results and pathological findings.

The biopsies had revealed cancer in two cores from the lower right side of the gland with a Gleason score of $3 + 4$. His prostate tumor was nonpalpable by DRE and was not visible by ultrasonic imaging or in a rectal coil MRI.

John had also undergone the reverse-transcriptase polymerase chain reaction (RT-PCR) for PSA assay. The test was negative.

Now that cancer was confirmed, John needed further guidance on his best course of action. We discussed treatment options at length. He consulted my surgical and radiation oncology colleagues as well.

Perhaps predictably, my surgical colleague recommended radical prostatectomy, and my radiation oncology colleague, while concurring that surgery was reasonable, felt that radiation was also a reasonable option. John was confused.

Treatment at that stage, I explained, was an investment for the future. The benefits of treatment in terms of years of life he gained from treatment would come years from now, maybe five or ten years, but some of the side effects would be immediate and could last the rest of his life.

While John considered this, I added, "You're only 58, John. You've got many good years ahead of you."

He nodded, weighing all the complex information the disease

had forced him to consider in the previous weeks. Based on what he'd learned, he felt the quality of his life was the most important thing to him, which might be better after treatment with radiation. Both his parents had died in their early sixties. "So," he said, "if I have ten more good years, I'll be happy."

Radiation might be easier to endure, I explained. However, if the cancer was contained within the prostate, surgery might offer a slightly higher cure rate over the long term.

"How much better?" John asked, grasping for solid data in the swirl of estimates and opinions. I couldn't quantify this estimate. The main factor in determining his likelihood of being cured wasn't the difference in effectiveness between treatments, but whether his cancer had already spread. I said, "Even though there is no indication of metastasis, there's a possibility the cancer has already spread." If surgery was better than radiation, I added, the difference in their effectiveness probably wouldn't affect him for five or possibly ten years.

John chose radiation therapy. He was treated with a standard course at a modern local radiation therapy center. He had predictable side effects, including minor bladder and bowel irritation. Over the course of months, John developed moderate sexual dysfunction. However, he heard about effective means to alleviate this problem through discussions with survivors in his prostate cancer support group. John opted for a combination of the vacuum device and injectable medications, which he alternates as circumstances vary. His level of sexual satisfaction has diminished only slightly.

Today, almost two years after diagnosis and treatment, John has a PSA of 0.5 ng/ml and a normal-feeling prostate. Every indication is that he is cured, although we will not be certain of this for years.

10

Metastatic Prostate Cancer I: Hormonal Therapy

Although being diagnosed with prostate cancer is frightening and treatment options can be bewildering, your confusion and fear may be most intense after a diagnosis of metastatic prostate cancer. Metastatic prostate cancer has spread by the lymphatics (lymph vessels) or the blood vessels from the prostate to other parts of the body. You might suffer a crushing sense of impending doom because medicine considers metastatic prostate cancer to be incurable. Some men who already feel that the disease has conquered them may be emotionally prepared to surrender.

The first question these men ask is often, "Doctor, how long do I have to live?" You should try to understand that this is a very difficult question for physicians to answer. First, doctors want and need to be honest and sincere; and we want to be supportive, but the generally unpredictable behavior of the disease, especially its elusive natural history, and its ability to take a much different course in men the same age make it difficult to decipher.

Another question that is asked that is certainly on the minds of many men is, "How much will I suffer?"

Most men do rebound emotionally. We are surprisingly resilient. And men are usually prepared to fight the disease. They will then ask, "What type of treatment do you recommend?"

The Diagnosis of Metastatic Prostate Cancer

The most conclusive evidence that prostate cancer has spread in your body comes from the radiographic imaging tests that your doctor will no doubt request you undergo. And the bone scan is the most important of these tests. Remember, a bone scan is not an X-ray; it is a test that locates areas of bone in which there is unusual metabolic activity. This activity is frequently due to cancer: bony metastases. The bone scan is a more sensitive test for metastasis from prostate cancer than is an X-ray. The scan is a painless procedure in which you are injected with a radioactive marker isotope that is absorbed by the living tissue of your bone. The scanner is something like a large Geiger counter; it detects the faint radioactive emissions from the absorbed marker isotope as you lie on the table beneath the scanner head. The image of these emissions can be printed as a type of photograph.

As I discussed earlier, when prostate cancer spreads to your bone, metastases most frequently form in the bones surrounding your pelvis, the lower spine, hips, or bones of the upper leg. You may have thought of bone as a solid lifeless structure similar to metal or plastic. But your bone is a living tissue, which on the microscopic level is anything but solid.

It is within the complex, near-microscopic honeycomb of living bone that prostate cancer metastases often seed themselves. Once this occurs, the treatment of prostate cancer is much more difficult. Medicine does not have the tools needed to destroy or remove all of the prostate cancer metastases from the entire human body.

The bone scan confirms the diagnosis of suspected metastatic disease — often prompted by very high PSA levels or by symptoms related to metastases in bone.

Due to several factors that we will detail in our discussion of bone pain, prostate cancer metastases cause an abnormal overgrowth called blastic bone change. This involves an overstimulation of bone-forming cells — osteoblasts — that becomes visible on the bone scan. More radioactive marker is absorbed in the areas of metastases than by normal bone. And these sites appear as characteristic dark spots on your bone scan.

However, all dark areas on your bone scan are not necessarily prostate cancer metastases. Arthritis — which most of us have as we age — can produce similar dark areas in your bone scan. Therefore, your radiologist and treating physician need to consider the full context of your bone scan, including the number and locations of lesions. They must also consider the likelihood of bone metastases as predicted by your PSA level. Remember that PSA is produced by prostate epithelial cells; the more cells, the higher the PSA. A very high PSA often indicates the presence of metastases, usually in bone. It is important to note, however, that a bone scan that shows no metastasis is not definitive, since the clumps of cells in metastases may not have grown to the point to produce changes that are visible on your bone scan. Unfortunately there is not a more sensitive test, including the the CT scan and MRI.

Plain-film X-rays may also be helpful. Abnormal blastic change may appear as unnaturally white areas, showing bone overgrowth we call sclerosis. In a similar way, MRI scans of a suspected area can be helpful to confirm or rule out metastases. However, some spots that are suspicious for cancer on the bone scan may not appear on your plain X-ray or MRI; therefore your doctor might call for a bone biopsy.

The CT scan is another diagnostic tool your doctor might use to confirm — or rule out — early metastatic disease. This computed tomography, as we already noted, is a computer-enhanced X-ray process that provides fairly detailed horizontal "slice" images of your body, which, unlike conventional X-rays, include both bone and soft tissue. CT scans of your pelvic region can reveal characteristic enlargement of the lymph nodes. The lymph nodes may also be enlarged in the back of your abdomen, the retroperitoneum. However, detecting lymph node enlargement on a CT scan is unusual. The entire range of findings from bone scans, CT scans, and other diagnostic X-rays provides what we call radiographic evidence of metastatic spread.

Other clinical evidence, particularly the PSA assay, can also be useful at this point. The higher your PSA, the greater the likelihood of metastasis. My concern increases with a PSA above 20 ng/ml. PSA levels above 50 ng/ml almost always indicate metastasis, whether or not I find it in a scan. Although a biopsy can provide proof through pathologic confirmation, radiographic evidence coupled with PSA levels is usually all your doctor needs to make this diagnosis.

If your radiographic findings are ambiguous (for instance, if your CT scan reveals lymph node enlargement), your doctor may suggest a lymphadenectomy (the surgical removal of certain pelvic lymph nodes) or a needle biopsy of a lymph node. The lymphadenectomy can be conducted either through conventional surgery (open pelvic surgery) or laparoscopic surgery. In the latter, the surgeons guide thin, flexible tube instruments by watching fiber-optic video images.

In less than one third of newly diagnosed prostate cancer cases, the cancer has already spread. This condition can sometimes be confirmed by bone or CT scan. Often, such men have no symptoms, but their physician recommends these scans because of a very elevated PSA level. Alternatively, sometimes your first realization of metastatic prostate cancer is pain in the bones, most often of your pelvis or back.

If the prostate cancer has spread to pelvic lymph nodes (the nodes near your prostate) but metastasis is not evident in your bone scans, your prognosis can be quite good. If this is your situation, your life expectancy might be five to ten years. If you are older, this means you might reach your normal life expectancy and die of other causes.

Unfortunately, treatment is not curative, although hormonal treatment will place you into remission. Ultimately, if you live long enough, the cancer may emerge in your bones after the effect of the hormone treatment has worn off.

General Characteristics of Metastatic Prostate Cancer

Be assured that most men achieve a remission when metastatic disease is treated. Your PSA assay and the bone scan are useful in charting this remission (regression and stabilization of disease) as well as recurrence (reassertment of disease). This means that your treatment can be adjusted to changing conditions when appropriate.

The second point you should remember is that metastatic prostate cancer does not usually progress with the speed of certain other cancers. Therefore, although metastatic prostate cancer is not presently curable, how long — and how well — one lives with metastatic disease varies greatly among individuals. If you're an older man with other medical problems, metastatic prostate cancer — although potentially life threatening — might not be the reason you die; it might not even be a major contributing factor. If you are in your 70s or 80s, for example, you might well succumb to cardiovascular disease that is unrelated to your cancer.

Metastatic Disease — Your Prognosis

Clinical research shows that the average survival following a diagnosis of metastatic prostate cancer in bone is almost three years. What do these stark figures mean to you? Half of the men with metastatic prostate cancer will die before three years, but half will survive longer. Remember, however, you are not a ballpark statistic; you're an individual. You may fit in anywhere on the curve. And, if you are a long-term survivor, a cure might come along in the future.

Where you fit on this continuum is difficult to determine due to uncertainty about a tumor's metastatic pattern and responsiveness to treatment. Most of the characteristics that predicted your tumor's growth behavior in the early stage are not useful in predicting behavior of the cancer once it has metastasized. This is most notable for the characteristic of cancer grade. The cancer's original grade tells you little about its behavior after it has spread.

A man's PSA level and trend are still useful predictors of response to treatment and survival. In general, the higher your PSA level, the more advanced your cancer is. For example, if you have a PSA of 25 ng/ml, usually you have less tumor than a level of 2,000 ng/ml, which no doubt signifies extensive metastatic involvement.

Your bone scans also provide important information. A fewer number of lesions (black spots representing tumor metastatic sites) in your bone is better than a large number of lesions. And your overall health — whether or not you have symptoms, whether you're energetic or frail — is a useful predictor of how you will fare.

The most important single variable among patients is the degree to which their cancer responds to hormonal therapy. You might have a long remission during hormonal therapy that lasts for years. If you have a less hormonally sensitive tumor, your remission will probably be less dramatic and shorter.

I tell people that there is always uncertainty and variability to response, but most men with metastatic disease can look forward to at least several years of good quality life.

"You have at least a couple of years before the situation changes," I explain to these men and their families. "It is important to get over this psychological hurdle, move on with your life, and structure it in a way that is best for you."

This is my advice to you: enjoy your remaining quality years, and prepare for the changes that may occur. You also must recognize your own mortality. If you are an older man and you've already made all the requisite legal and financial arrangements for your final years, this advice is not so critical. But if you're younger, this frank advice can be a shock. However, try to take comfort in the knowledge that you can probably look forward to several years of good quality of life during the remission.

Variables in Hormonal Therapy

After hormonal therapy is initiated, your androgen supply to prostate cancer cells is effectively shut off. When this occurs, cells die by undergoing a process called programmed cell death, or apoptosis. Some cells remain dormant and do not die. The proportion of cells that die determines the success of your therapy. Cancer cells that are less responsive or less sensitive to hormonal therapy are ultimately the ones that go on to emerge if you endure a relapse.

In prostate cancer, some of the malignant cells will be more dependent than others on male hormones (androgens). These male hormones are said to be "mitogenic," that is, androgens are needed for the mitosis or reproduction of the prostate cancer cells. I often use the analogy that androgens are essentially the food needed for the survival and growth of most prostate cancer cells. And the proportion of androgen-dependent cells in the metastases is the key factor in the effectiveness of your hormonal treatment.

You should note that hormonal therapy is somewhat of a misnomer, for the treatments commonly used are not hormones per se, but rather hormone blockers or drug treatments that reduce the effect of hormones. The one exception is estrogens such as diethylstilbestrol (DES) — a female hormone.

Hormonal therapy works by either removing your supply of androgen or by blocking the effects of androgens. There are several ways of accomplishing this endpoint: by surgical means, for example, the removal of the testicles (bilateral orchiectomy), or through the use of medication to decrease production of the principal male hormone, testosterone.

A large percentage of prostate cancers are quite hormonally sensitive. The malignant cells in these metastatic cancers cannot reproduce very well without the presence of androgens. Therefore, when male hormones are withdrawn, by whatever means, you go into a remission.

After your hormonal therapy, you may have a relatively brief remission before the disease inevitably advances again. This is because most of the cancer cells were relatively hormonally insensitive.

Hormonal Therapy: When Should I Be Treated?

There is some controversy as to when to begin hormonal therapy following a diagnosis of metastatic disease.

Traditionally, hormonal treatment was not started until symptoms appeared. But in recent years many physicians and patients have opted for hormonal therapy much earlier in the course of the disease. This shift has occurred not as a result of definitive research but rather as a change in philosophical approach that many American physicians took toward prostate cancer by treating metastatic disease more aggressively.

An important factor in this treatment shift is the effort to alleviate the anxiety one feels about living with cancer that is not being treated. Hormonal therapy is being offered more frequently to men with stage D1 prostate cancer, despite the fact that the proven benefits of treatment with regard to length of survival remain undocumented.

If you have metastatic prostate cancer, these are your two most important questions:

- How long will I live with this disease?
- What will my quality of life be during these years?

Hormonal therapy probably does have an impact on the length of your life after diagnosis and treatment — although that has not yet been documented.

Doctors have also learned from experience that hormonal therapy is a good treatment for men with symptoms. Any physician who has treated such men knows that hormonal therapy will help alleviate pain and thus have a positive effect on your quality of life. The hormonal approach to treatment reduces your pain that comes from the bone metastases because it kills many of the cancer cells in those sites.

When to Begin Hormonal Therapy

Your doctor may take the traditional view that hormonal therapy should be reserved until you experience symptoms, since hormonal therapy alleviates pain as opposed to curing the disease. In other words, your doctor is putting more stock in the enhancement of quality of life than in the treatment's yet unproven role in prolonging your survival if used early. However, another doctor might argue for early institution of hormonal therapy because this might delay the onset of your symptoms and thus enhance your quality of life even more.

The potential risks and benefits of your treatment become more pressing in the later stages of the disease. Then the critical question is, What are the chances that a specific treatment will actually help me?

With metastatic prostate cancer, the benefit of a specific treatment has to be weighed in terms of increased life expectancy and enhanced quality of life for the duration of your life. You should be prepared to ask your doctor about the benefit of any treatment at every stage of the disease.

You may be among those men who have great difficulty living with a cancer that is not being treated. For you, intervention through some form of treatment becomes an important element in your quality of life. You and your physician should frankly discuss all the advantages and the disadvantages, physical and psychological, to determine the optimal time to start hormonal treatment.

If you have metastatic prostate cancer documented by bone scan or CT scan, I recommend initiating hormonal therapy. Because it is generally only a matter of months until symptoms occur after such a diagnosis, it is beneficial if your symptoms can be avoided or at least delayed.

If you do not have radiographic confirmation of metastasis but you have earlier metastatic disease — stage D1 or detectable and rising PSA levels after surgery or radiation therapy — talk over your treatment options thoroughly with your doctor.

Remember, the advantage of the proactive approach is the delay of the onset of symptoms. The disadvantage of beginning hormonal therapy if you do not have symptoms is that you are committed to lifelong therapy, which has the side effects of sexual impotence and hot flashes. If you readily accept these disadvantages, go ahead and start hormonal therapy.

Types of Hormonal Therapy

Don't confuse hormonal therapy with chemotherapy. They are distinctly different forms of therapy. Remember, hormonal therapy removes the metabolic food your prostate cancer cells need to survive and grow. Many of these cells die or remain dormant. Chemotherapy drugs are toxic directly to the cells through a variety of ways relating to their metabolism.

Hormonal therapy for advanced or metastatic prostate cancer is palliative treatment: it alleviates symptoms and may prolong life expectancy without bringing a cure. The word palliate comes from the Latin word *pallium,* a cloak. Hormonal therapy cloaks, or covers, symptoms (pain) but does not cure them. Although hormonal therapy may improve quality of life and may even increase your life expectancy, the treatment rarely rids your body of the disease. However, a cloak can provide great comfort, and in this regard palliation is quite successful.

Hormonal therapy almost always brings a remission — a respite, not a cure. Ultimately, clones of the cancer cells will emerge that are not sensitive to the androgen ablation that brought the original remission. When this occurs, you'll need additional treatment.

Hormonal Therapy: Practical Aspects

Hormonal therapy removes the male hormone from your body through a variety of techniques.

Male hormones, or androgens, are produced largely in the testicles in the form of testosterone. Your body converts this into another androgen called dihydrotestosterone (DHT). Testosterone and its biproduct act as metabolic stimulants for your prostate cancer cells. However, a proportion of the male hormone circulating in your blood is not derived from the testicles, but is produced in the adrenal glands adjacent to your kidneys. The amount of male hormone (predominately androstenedrone and dehydroepiandrosterone) derived from the adrenal glands varies among individuals and during the course of the disease in any particular patient. But your adrenal androgens average around 10 percent of the total androgen in your blood.

Orchiectomy

The traditional method of stopping male hormone production is surgical castration, the removal of both testicles, a procedure called a bilateral orchiectomy. This relatively minor operation removes the principal source of testosterone.

The advantage of orchiectomy is that it is a one-time treatment. After the procedure, you can continue your life without the disruption of ongoing regular treatment. You must recognize, however, that this is an irreversible step: permanent sexual impotence ensues. I recommend orchiectomy for men who know their options, have no psychological difficulties with this procedure, and who want to live their remaining years with as few disruptions as possible.

Medical Therapy

Nonsurgical androgen suppression has long been used to manage metastatic prostate cancer. Until recently, this usually involved administering an estrogen such as diethylstilbestrol (DES), similar to the estrogen replacement prescribed for many postmenopausal women. DES therapy for prostate cancer is easy to use — one to three pills daily — and is inexpensive.

Because of its higher rate of cardiovascular side effects, it must be used judiciously. Indeed, DES treatment is now unusual because the associated risk of heart problems and blood clots, although small, precludes its use for many older patients. DES also has the side effect of breast enlargement and tenderness.

DES has largely been replaced by a newer nonsurgical form of hormonal treatment, called luteinizing hormone-releasing hormone (LH-RH) blockers, or analogs.[1] Your doctor might prescribe the forms of these drugs that are available commercially, leuprolide (Lupron) or gosereline (Zoladex). These compounds act as chemical messengers that influence the pituitary gland at the base of your brain. The LH-RH blockers prevent your pituitary from releasing a hormone that triggers testosterone secretion in your testicles. With this pituitary hormone suppressed, your testicular production of male hormones almost completely ceases. By suppressing testosterone levels, this drug treatment is equally as effective as orchiectomy in terms of hindering tumor activity.

Therapy with LH-RH analog requires monthly visits to your doctor for shots of the drug. Preparations are now available; their duration is three months. They are equally effective. The shot causes minimal discomfort because the "depot" medication has to be injected either into a thick muscle of your buttock or abdomen (in the case of Lupron) or as a pellet into the tissue beneath the skin. You can minimize the discomfort by using some topical anesthetic or numbing medicine before the injection. This drug therapy is currently very expensive, with the required monthly treatment costing as much as $400 for the medication alone. Medicare and private insurers pay for LH-RH medication, provided you have been diagnosed with metastatic prostate cancer. LH-RH therapy is the alternative of choice if you do not want to undergo what you might see as a drastic step in the form of an orchiectomy.

These two forms of hormonal therapy, orchiectomy and LH-RH blockers, are equivalent: they both achieve a near-total reduction of your testicular testosterone and they are equivalent with regard to efficacy. This hormonal reduction will most likely bring you a remission of disease.

If you have pain symptoms, you will experience significant relief through hormonal therapy. There will usually be a decrease in your PSA level and perhaps an improvement in your bone scan or other radiographic evidence of disease. The duration of your positive response to hormonal therapy (remission) is highly variable. Research indicates the average remission duration is about two years; however, it varies greatly from person to person. When the remission is over, you will need other forms of treatment. It is probable that hormonal therapy will play a role in extending your life expectancy.

Hormonal Therapy: Side Effects

Both orchiectomy and LH-RH therapy have similar side effects, principally the loss of sex drive, and sexual impotence. You should recognize that this is a different condition than the sexual dysfunction resulting from radical prostatectomy or radiation therapy, in which you usually retain your normal sex drive but can experience problems with achieving erection. Because male sex drive is principally controlled by androgens and their removal is the goal of hormonal therapy, loss of your libido (sex drive) is an unfortunate side effect of this therapy. Suspending LH-RH analogs will allow testosterone levels — and libido — to return, but continual therapy is generally recommended indefinitely. (We will discuss intermittent hormone therapy later in this chapter.)

Most men treated with orchiectomy or LH-RH blockers develop hot flashes, a common side effect of hormonal therapy. Typically, a sudden, brief period of warmth is followed by profuse sweating. These hot flashes are similar to the discomfort experienced by menopausal women. The frequency of this side effect varies among men, but only occasionally becomes very distressing. If it does, you may take low doses of DES, another hormonal medication called megastrol acetate (sold as Megace), or a medication called Clonidine, delivered by a skin patch. Though hot flashes are common, relatively few of my patients have required treatment for them.

Remember, the choice of either orchiectomy or LH-RH is based on your personal desire, not medical factors. Both forms of treatment are equally effective.

If you are uncertain as to which treatment is best for you, I usually recommend LH-RH hormonal therapy until you make your final decision.

Case History: Orchiectomy

Grant C., age 78, is a widower. He lives with a daughter and son-in-law, and he devotes much of his time to his retirement hobby, cabinet-making. He went to his family doctor in western Massachusetts, complaining of low back pain, which he thought was due to heavy lifting in his workshop.

Grant's doctor prescribed analgesics, but these drugs did not relieve the pain. His doctor then ordered a bone scan, which revealed dark-spot abnormalities in Grant's lower spine, pelvic bones, ribs, and the long bones of his upper legs. These abnormalities suggested bone metastases.

Grant underwent a prostate cancer evaluation. His PSA was extremely elevated: 367 ng/ml. His prostate was enlarged but contained no obvious hard nodules. The sextant biopsy was positive in three of the six cores, with a Gleason score of $4 + 4 = 8$. This suggested a potentially aggressive tumor, which would account for the almost certain metastatic spread of disease.

When I consulted with Grant, he was accompanied by his daughter and son-in-law, who were clearly distraught over his diagnosis. Grant, a confident man who had overcome the hardships of the Great Depression and World War II, was more accepting.

"The main thing is the pain," he explained. "I just want to be able to get back in the shop and finish some projects." He added that he wanted the simplest possible treatment that would allow him to return to his normal life.

I recommended orchiectomy. It was simple, I explained; it was safe, and it was over in one visit.

"That's the way we'll go," Grant said. He added with a smile, "Sex drive isn't one of my big priorities right now."

One month after the outpatient surgery, Grant returned to my clinic. There was better color to his face and a firmer tone to his voice. "The pain is completely gone," he announced. This simple form of hormonal treatment was a wise choice for Grant.

Antiandrogen Therapy

Another form of hormonal treatment you should consider is antiandrogen therapy. Antiandrogens are chemicals that do not stop the production of your male hormone, but rather block the effect of androgens on prostate tissue at the cellular or molecular level. These compounds prevent your testosterone and dihydrotestosterone from stimulating the growth of prostate cells, including those malignant cells present in your prostate cancer metastases.

The most commonly used antiandrogens with proven benefit are flutamide (Eulexin) and bicalutamide (Casodex). Some studies have indicated that when used in conjunction with either an orchiectomy or LH-RH therapy, these types of drugs prolong the hormonal remission period. Furthermore, although not all the studies agree, there has also been some encouraging research indicating this combination of therapies might actually prolong your survival when compared to the use of LH-RH blockers or orchiectomy used alone.

Ask your doctor about using flutamide or bicalutamide in conjunction with orchiectomy or LH-RH analog. You might start these drugs one week before beginning your LH-RH analog in order to block an uncommon but possible testosterone-level flare-up, a reaction to the introduction of LH-RH therapy.

Flutamide may give you diarrhea, which is often difficult to treat unless the dose of the drug is diminished or stopped. This occurs in about 10 to 15 percent of the men using flutamide. The antiandrogen may also cause liver function problems, usually minor, so your physician should check your liver function tests periodically for rare but potentially serious liver disruption. Bicalutamide, which is relatively new, has the potential advantage of its single daily dose compared to flutamide (taken three times a day), as well as a probable lower incidence of diarrhea.

Newer Investigational Options for Hormonal Therapy

Ask your doctor about the experimental treatment programs under way at medical centers across the country. Two interesting approaches are potency-sparing hormonal therapy and intermittent hormonal therapy.

Research on potency-sparing hormonal therapy is based on the principle that antiandrogens usually allow you to retain your sex drive while being treated because they do not disrupt your production of testosterone, which controls sex drive, but rather interfere with the attachment of the male hormone to receptors in prostate cells. Some of this promising research has used an antiandrogen such as flutamide or bicalutamide alone. Another approach is to use one of these antiandrogens in conjunction with a drug called finasteride (brand name Proscar), which inhibits an enzyme (5-alpha reductase) that your prostate cells (either benign or malignant) need to convert your testosterone into dihydrotestosterone.

Obviously, retaining sex drive is an important consideration for many of you, and this potency-sparing approach to hormonal therapy now being studied promises to provide you an important quality-of-life alternative to standard therapy. However, from a survival standpoint, this treatment has not yet been compared with conventional hormonal therapy. You should definitely discuss this option with your doctor.

You might consider another experimental approach, intermittent hormonal therapy. As noted, prostate cancer contains cells that have differing degrees of dependence on male hormones (androgens). When your androgens are reduced either through orchiectomy or LH-RH analog therapy, the most androgen-dependent cells die and those that are less dependent survive and ultimately multiply.

The rationale behind intermittent treatment is that the presence of androgen-sensitive cells might actually inhibit the growth of insensitive clones, either by vying for the same metabolic substances or by directly inhibiting their growth. Eradicating sensitive clones through uninterrupted hormonal therapy might actually permit the uncontrolled growth of hormone insensitive prostate cancer cells. So, if you periodically interrupt your LH-RH hormonal therapy, you might actually reduce the proportion of uncontrollable cancer cells in your tumor. This approach is still unproven, but ask your doctor if it is appropriate for you.[2]

Research also promises to make available different preparations of LH-RH analogs. Instead of the current monthly treatment, we may soon be able to inject once every three months.

Research is also addressing LH-RH vaccines that block the production of luteinizing hormones in the pituitary gland. This approach would require you to have a few initial injections followed by periodic boosters. The vaccine technique looks promising because it eliminates the need for both orchiectomy and monthly injections.

Measuring the Success of Hormonal Therapy

As discussed, the interpretation of PSA levels differs for different clinical situations. A PSA level of say 6.0 ng/ml means something different if you have just had a PSA test for screening than if you have received radiation or have undergone a radical prostatectomy. And the significance of PSA level is also different if you have been treated with hormonal therapy.

As is the case following radical prostatectomy and radiation therapy, hormonal therapy should cause a drop in your PSA level. Periodic PSA determinations will help chart the course of your hormonal therapy. It may take months, however, for your PSA to reach its lowest point. As a general rule, the lower your PSA drops, the more effective has been the treatment.

Once your PSA has decreased to its lowest level, it should remain stable, sometimes with minor fluctuations. I have found that while some men are satisfied knowing that they have been treated and that the cancer is going into remission, most men want to know the direction in which their PSA level is going. My advice is to move on with your life and allow your physician to track the course. Some patients will tell me, "Let me know when I need to know." Others must know everything, and that's all right, too. In general, your PSA can be checked every few months during hormonal therapy.

One's PSA level is the most sensitive and earliest indicator of relapse when undergoing hormonal therapy. A rising trend in your PSA level will in all likelihood come before clinically evident recurrence or the onset of symptoms. That is to say, an increasing PSA level will usually predate symptoms of bone pain or radiographic evidence (bone or CT scans). So there is usually no need for bone scans or CT scans following hormonal therapy until your PSA begins to climb.

Again, the advent of the PSA assay has changed the way medicine manages prostate cancer. In the past, after you underwent hormonal therapy and your symptoms were alleviated, you would remain in remission until symptoms returned. Now, however, with the PSA assay available, it is possible to detect recurrence before you feel symptoms.

The knowledge that your prostate cancer is recurring often creates anxiety in both you and your doctor. Therefore, if you are a metastatic prostate cancer patient, try to achieve an honest dialogue with your physician regarding your prognosis. This is dependent on multiple factors, including the extent of metastatic spread and the apparent sensitivity of the cancer's cells to hormonal deprivation, once the treatment has begun.

In Chapter 11, we will discuss the courses of treatment of prostate cancer when the disease recurs following hormonal therapy.

Case History: Treating the Patient after an Unsuccessful Radical Prostatectomy

Doug C. was 58 in 1993, at the pinnacle of a successful career with a communications corporation. He underwent a physical examination that included a PSA assay. His level was high: 13.0 ng/ml. Because he had no signs or symptoms of BPH or prostatitis, his family physician was immediately suspicious of prostate cancer. The physician recommended a full workup for prostate cancer, including a biopsy.

Because Doug experienced no symptoms whatsoever, he decided against the biopsy, despite his physician's advice. He also avoided taking another PSA assay for the next six months. "I deluded myself," Doug now admits. "I was in denial and didn't want to face the prospect of cancer."

He chose to consult the urologist to whom his family physician had originally referred him. His next PSA was higher: 15.0 ng/ml. Doug underwent a biopsy. He recounts, "It was positive in two of six cores. I had never received such negative news in my life."

The pathological grade of the tumor was Gleason score 3 + 4. The ultrasonic imaging, CT scan, and bone scan were slightly ambiguous but suggestive that the cancer had not spread beyond the confines of the prostate.

Medical friends recommended that Doug visit the Dana-Farber Cancer Institute for a consultation. I met Doug in our clinic, where patients receive advice from urologists and radiation and medical oncologists.

I first saw Doug several weeks after his biopsy. The PSA he'd undergone at Dana-Farber also rendered a level of 15.0 ng/ml. I suggested that he undergo an MRI because the PSA was particularly high and he was considering surgery. The MRI showed no evidence of extracapsular extension and no seminal vesicle involvement. Based on this evidence, and after discussion among my colleagues and then with Doug — who fully understood the risks and potential benefits of treatment — we recommended radical prostatectomy. Doug concurred.

During the procedure, the surgeon removed a representative sampling of pelvic lymph nodes for immediate frozen-section biopsy. The results revealed that Doug's cancer had spread to several of these lymph nodes. The surgeon did not complete the radical prostatectomy, but instead closed the incision.

It was now established that Doug had early metastatic prostate cancer: malignant cells had escaped from the primary tumor site in his prostate through the lymphatic system and undoubtedly had spread elsewhere in his body. These malignant seeds had not yet grown to significant metastases that could be detected on a bone scan or CT scan.

This information put Doug in a gray zone. If he had obvious bone metastases, I would have strongly recommended hormonal therapy. But he had no symptoms and showed no pathological evidence of metastatic spread beyond the pelvic lymph nodes. And since he was a vigorous, sexually active man in his late fifties, the complete loss of libido inherent to standard hormonal therapy seemed unacceptable to Doug and his wife. But they felt strongly that they needed to proceed with some form of treatment; the anxiety of not doing anything was too great.

I suggested that Doug consider participating in a research

study, or protocol, of potency-sparing therapy involving a combination of the 5-alpha reductase inhibitor finasteride (Proscar) with the antiandrogen flutamide (Eulexin). This protocol, or experimental trial, was being conducted at Dana-Farber. Some of the patients in the study had case histories similar to Doug's.

I explained to Doug that the therapy is based on the theory that the antiandrogen flutamide (Eulexin) prevents circulating androgens from having a stimulating effect on prostate cancer cells, while the 5-alpha reductase inhibitor finasteride (Proscar) prevents the conversion of testosterone into dihydrotestosterone, the most potent stimulator of prostate cancer cell growth.

Those of us involved with this study were confident that the combined therapy would dampen the metabolic activity of prostate epithelial cells throughout the patients' bodies, and perhaps delay the onset of clinically significant metastatic cancer. The preservation of sex drive, which was always lost in standard hormonal therapy, was an attractive factor in this treatment.

Several months into the experimental treatment, Doug had no side effects. His PSA had dropped to undetectable levels. However, he went through a period of depression following the confirmation that the disease had spread beyond the prostate. He became preoccupied with death; morbid thoughts arose whenever words such as "impending" or "imminent" came up in normal conversation. Some days he simply sat by a window in his house, staring blankly at the trees and waiting for five o'clock to arrive, when he could mix his first martini with some degree of self-respect. He was convinced the prostate cancer was spreading rapidly in his system and would quickly kill him.

Doug's primary care physician prescribed antidepressant medications. After a couple of months, he emerged from the depression. In addition to the antidepressants, one of the factors involved with recovery of emotional well-being was learning the results of his ongoing examinations: his PSA stayed low and his DRE, which was initially abnormal, had returned to normal, the result of the combined flutamide and finasteride therapy.

Another contributing factor to Doug's recovery from depression was his friendship with a man who is in the final stages of metastatic colon cancer. Although this man's condition was more serious than Doug's, his attitude remained positive and his spirits high. Moreover, Doug's friend has maintained a reasonable quality of life for three years while battling his cancer.

"I saw him as a kind of mirror image," Doug told me recently. "And I realized that I had not come even close to his condition. So, I knew I had a lot of good years left."

Because Doug remains symptom free, it is easier for him to recognize that the metastatic disease has not yet significantly advanced. He has plenty of energy and now walks almost five miles every day. "I've never felt healthier or more full of life," Doug told me.

Indeed, he has decided to make the most of his life. He is now retired and is free of the daily stress of corporate life. He has acquired the ability to relish the moment, to take pleasure in the simple activities of daily life. "I have a definite sense of the *now,*" he explains.

On his daily walks he makes sure to pass through the Boston Public Garden, where he literally stops to smell the flowers and to chat with the gardeners.

"I treasure my grandchildren," Doug says. Before his diagnosis of prostate cancer, he had always thought he had many years to devote to each grandchild. Now he realizes that spending time with them is more important than almost anything else. He now attends school recitals and sporting events he might have missed in the past.

I told Doug that what he had gone through was perhaps a more extreme version of the battering on the emotional rollercoaster that most men and their families experience after the diagnosis of prostate cancer.

Doug agreed. "It's one thing to get older," he said. "But it's another thing altogether to experience for the first time the *wall* of mortality. This disease has made me face the years I have left and use them well."

I am currently monitoring Doug's progress.

11

Metastatic Prostate Cancer II: When Hormonal Therapy Fails

Introduction

Although metastatic prostate cancer cannot be cured with today's medical technology, your doctors can help you to optimize the quality of your life and perhaps prolong your life. If you have metastatic disease, I am sure you are coming to terms with this reality.

In this section, I'll try to offer you all the resources available to me to help you cope with and adjust to your disease. I will try to provide information that will assist you and your doctor to better care for your mind as well as your body. I strive to coordinate my patients' care, to be their advocate and friend, and to provide emotional support. Since I know what lies ahead, I try to be their scout along their treatment path. I hope to aid you in a similar way.

You should not be pessimistic about your treatment options if the illness is no longer responsive to hormonal therapy. But you should also recognize that an activist treatment approach must be conducted within the parameters of realistic goals, devoid of false expectations, and with a careful balance between the risk and benefit of treatment.

Any treatment plan developed at the advanced stage of cancer should contain a range of specific options designed to maintain or improve your quality of life. You can meet this goal through a carefully conceived and executed program of comprehensive specialized care, which includes medical, surgical, and radiation oncologists and specialized nursing and psychosocial support.

When hormonal therapy stops working, you are in the hormone refractory phase of the disease, or are said to have "hormone insensitive" metastatic prostate cancer. Whatever the terminology used, the condition is the same. As you approach this phase of prostate cancer, you can still find treatments that might bring a respite in your disease or a remission. If conventional therapy has failed, you might seek out experimental treatments.

I noted earlier that hormonal therapy sometimes remains an effective palliative treatment until the end of a man's life, with some men ultimately dying of diseases unrelated to prostate cancer. For many advanced prostate cancer patients, however, the disease follows a different course. At some point after the initiation of hormonal therapy the PSA begins to rise, and the bone scan or CT scan also may show that the remission period has ended, which means that the progress of the disease has resumed.

In any malignant prostate tumor (including its metastases), a proportion of the cancerous cells are dependent on male hormones (androgens) for their growth and replication. Thus, hormone ablation or deprivation therapy by whatever means starves these cells of a critical metabolic "food." Without androgens, most of these hormone-dependent cells cannot flourish and they eventually disappear.

Unfortunately, cells and the tumors that comprise them develop clever ways of overcoming the absence of androgen. Some cells mutate so that they can grow in very low levels of androgen, while others devise ways to grow without androgen at all. It appears that these cells and the tumors that comprise them are androgen independent, or hormone refractory. Therefore, the malignancy becomes refractory — not responsive to — hormonal deprivation. You might find this concept confusing. The surviving cancer cells do not suddenly become resistant to hormone deprivation. The mutated cells that emerge existed prior to hormonal therapy but developed more extensively over time. Suffice it to say that during the hormone refractory stage of prostate cancer, most of the remaining malignant cells cannot be kept under control by androgen deprivation.

After the failure of hormonal therapy, the hormone refractory portion of prostate cancer cells grows, both in the original tumor (if still extant) and its metastases. Generally the PSA levels reflect this by showing a rising trend. Also, metastatic sites may begin to appear (or reappear) in bone scans. Often the rising PSA trend, after a sharp decline during successful hormonal therapy, is the first indication that this treatment is no longer effective. Positive bone scans will sometimes coincide with this rise in PSA, but will rarely precede it.

There is not yet a single, well-established therapeutic approach that all physicians follow when metastatic prostate cancer reaches this point. When PSA, clinical (the patient's own symptoms), and radiographic evidence clearly indicate that hormonal therapy has failed, doctors do not have any one standard approach to follow in managing the disease. At this stage you need a doctor you can rely on who will focus on your total care, an advocate to manage your treatment plan. Some men will continue under the care of their urologist or radiation oncologist if they have established a good rapport with them. Some turn to their primary care physician or internist; others seek the care of a medical oncologist.

Those who turn to medical oncologists often find that although my colleagues and I don't have a single gold-standard treatment available for everyone, we are confident that we can help you pursue your goal — to optimize your quality of life and perhaps extend your survival.

Approaches to Hormone Refractory Prostate Cancer

How should you proceed if your prostate cancer no longer responds to hormonal therapy?

The first point in this treatment approach is to verify whether or not your hormonal therapy is indeed no longer working. By definition, this means that we need to find out if, despite low levels of testosterone, your tumor is progressing. Remember, with orchiectomy and LH-RH antagonists at appropriate doses, testosterone levels are very low. But in other forms of treatment, such as estrogen therapy, the testosterone level may not be low; therefore, your testosterone level should be checked. The fact that the tumor is progressing is most reliably indicated by a rise in your PSA, which is not directly related to testosterone levels. Although there may be fluctuations in your PSA, a steady rise is unequivocal evidence.

The second part of the assessment is checking for symptoms. This may include general symptoms such as fatigue and loss of appetite or specific symptoms such as bone pain or difficulty urinating. My approach to men without symptoms is to alleviate their anxiety and to establish a plan. I explain that there are two approaches: treat the cancer only when symptoms occur, or treat it early, before symptoms occur.

Bear in mind that the major objective of treatment is to maintain a good quality of life as long as possible. Although treatment may also prolong life, it is difficult to be certain of this in any individual. Quality time is the most important factor. Some people may wait if they are feeling well, while others feel the need to do something proactive for their peace of mind, which may improve the quality of their life.

If you have symptoms, there is a two-pronged approach. The first tactic is symptom management, which may include pain relief, dietary consultation, and psychosocial assessment and support. The second tactic is anticancer therapy, which may be localized therapy (treating a specific area), such as bone irradiation, or systemic therapy (treating the entire body), such as chemotherapy.

After assessment, I listen carefully to my patient's goals, to what is most important to him and his family. Together we form a plan. I make sure that we all understand the plan is always flexible, subject to change.

The Issue of Pain

When you discuss tactics for treating advanced prostate cancer with your doctor, your early conversations may address the issue of pain. The threat of severe, chronic pain in metastatic cancer is undoubtedly one of the greatest fears you and your family must endure as you confront the disease. This fear contains a major component of uncertainty. You don't know how devastating the pain might be, but you assume the worst. Fear may arise during the symptom-free period preceding the onset of metastatic pain.

Rest assured that medicine will control the pain of your prostate cancer, reducing it to manageable, if not insignificant, proportions. You do not have to and should not suffer through the final phases of the disease under the unacceptable burden of severe pain.

You and your physician must work together closely on this critical aspect of treatment. If you are among the very few individuals in whom pain is difficult to manage, you should consult physicians who specialize in pain control. Accurately describe the nature (sharp, dull, constant, intermittent) and severity of your pain so that your doctor will have an adequate picture. Then he or she can better determine the exact causes of the pain and treat you more effectively.

Your family also has a major role to play. If you and your family understand the processes through which metastatic prostate cancer causes pain, you will be more successful in treating it.

Analyzing Metastatic Pain

First of all, not all pain that occurs in a patient with prostate cancer is caused by the cancer. We all have a variety of aches and pains that come and go. Many people have arthritis, for example, which may cause pain. Pain that persists for several days should be brought to your doctor's attention. Pain is a symptom of specific physiological processes. Oncologists are trained to link certain types of pain with their root causes. But before we can analyze the pain and treat it correctly, we must understand exactly what you are experiencing. This is not always easy because we all have different perceptions of pain and different levels of tolerance.

I frequently ask my patients to keep a regular pain diary, and I urge you to do the same. In this notebook you should write down the time you experience pain, its quality, its severity, and location, as well as any relationship to physical activity. A typical pain diary entry might read: "8:30 A.M., dull achy pain in the lower back. Pain began after climbing stairs. Pain lasted for two hours." The severity scale that we use ranges from one to ten. Such a pain diary is an effective way to communicate the nature and severity of your pain to your physician.

By reviewing your X-rays and bone scans, your doctor can check the location and the degree of metastatic involvement, as well as judge whether your symptoms point toward more serious neurological impairment. Thus, tracking pain can help your physician keep one step ahead of the problem by tailoring treatment options to match your symptoms.

Remember that medicine has developed adequate tools to control pain for the vast majority of metastatic prostate cancer patients. These include radiation therapy (both localized external beam and systemic radiopharmaceuticals), lesser analgesics, and narcotics.

Given this pain-fighting arsenal, the worst possible course you can take is to stoically battle your pain without communicating the problem to your physicians or nurses. A general principle of pain treatment is that it's easier to treat pain in a preventive fashion when it is mild than to treat it after it has become severe.

There is another advantage to preventing pain: you can dismiss the nagging reminder of the cancer's presence. Many advanced prostate cancer patients suffer a psychological blow when they first experience significant pain from metastases. They might say,

"The pain has begun. I'm losing the battle." This psychological trauma can trigger a sense of hopelessness and diminish your will to prevail. If you and your physician address pain management, you will alleviate this despair and minimize the severe pain itself.

The Mechanisms of Metastatic Bone Pain

Prostate cancer cells spread from the primary tumor in two ways. The first way is through the lymphatic channels that drain your pelvic cavity. The appearance of cancerous cells in the pelvic lymph nodes is a definitive marker of metastatic disease. The second route that metastatic prostate cancer seeds follow is the venous channels that drain blood from the pelvic area.

Microscopic clumps of cancer cells carried by the veins tend to preferentially take root in bone marrow, usually within the bones in proximity to your pelvic cavity: the lumbar spine, the pelvic bones themselves, or the long bones of your upper legs. Oncologists are not yet certain why this pattern of metastatic spread occurs. However, we believe that there is some biological factor in the marrow of bones that is conducive to the establishment of prostate cancer metastases.

Most of us picture bone marrow as the gel found in the central cavity of long bones. In actuality, marrow channels permeate most bone tissue in an irregular honeycomb (this is visible under low microscopic power). In this complex maze of marrow channels, prostate cancer metastases become established and eventually grow to significant mass.

Metastases first impact the surrounding bone tissue by causing physiological change at the cellular level. Chemicals secreted by the metastases stimulate both unnatural bone growth and bone destruction. Generally, there is an imbalance toward abnormal new bone formation around the growing metastases. This new bone tissue is simultaneously overly dense and weaker than normal bone. You'll remember that we call this abnormal overgrowth "blastic" bone change. It appears as whiter areas (richer in mineral) on a plain-film bone X-ray. When your doctors compare these X-ray views to the darker metastatic spots on your bone scan, there is usually a positional overlap.

The blastic overgrowth in the confined marrow channels, as well as the actual swelling mass of tumor, produces pressure. This can cause pain because the surface of your bones is laced with nerve fibers.

The other type of metastatic cancer damage to bone is destructive. Bone can become riddled with holes, a process that undermines the integrity of important structural bones of your legs, hips, and spine. This form of metastatic bone destruction is called "lytic" change. Lytic change does not appear on bone scans, in which the emitting radioisotope markers are absorbed by blastic overgrowth. Therefore, plain-film bone X-rays are an important diagnostic tool if lytic change is suspected. Fortunately, it is relatively unusual in prostate cancer.

Beyond actual physical encroachment on nerve fibers, metastatic prostate cancer might also produce pain through a complex biochemical process. Tumor cells in close proximity to nerve fibers secrete chemicals that cause these nerves to fire in patterns that produce pain.

Pain may arise directly at the site of metastatic bone involvement or may occur at some distance from the site in a process called "referred pain." This happens when tumor or blastic bone growth physically compresses your nerves, especially those that pass through relatively narrow bone channels, as in your spine. Referred pain may be constant or intermittent, depending on such factors as physical activity and body position.

Medications for Pain

Throughout the course of your disease, pain relieving medications are available to you in a wide variety of forms and strengths. There is no benefit in your delaying the use of pain medications based on the ungrounded fear that they might become ineffective later, when your pain can become more severe. These medications cover a broad spectrum of potency, and most can be used in doses that are safe and adequate in bringing relief.

All types of metastatic pain are not the same. You might experience a general ache that does not have a specific site of focus. Stiffness in a limb or in the neck and back is another way pain manifests itself. For these symptoms, relatively mild medications are sufficient. Severe localized pain requires stronger pain relief drugs, however.

On an ascending order of effect, pain relief medications begin with nonprescription analgesics such as acetaminophen (Tylenol) and nonsteroidal anti-inflammatory drugs (NSAIDs). These include aspirin and ibuprofen (Advil, Motrin, Nuprin). Other NSAIDs formerly only available under prescription, such as Anaprox (naproxen sodium), are also becoming available over the counter.

Steroidal anti-inflammatory drugs, such as hydrocortisone, are also often useful in treating painful flare-ups. Again, when you are able to describe accurately the nature and duration of your pain, your physician is better able to determine its cause and offer combinations of medications that bring relief.

The next step on the pain relief scale is narcotic analgesics. The mildest narcotic analgesic that I prescribe is codeine, generally in combination with acetaminophen (Tylenol #3). Synthetic opiates such as Percodan (oxycodone) have a greater analgesic effect. But bear in mind that NSAIDs may complement these drugs' effect and can frequently be used simultaneously. Ask your doctor about such combination therapies.

Persistent and severe pain usually requires narcotic therapy. Sustained release morphine preparations such as MS Contin or Duramorph, which act over long periods of time, are most useful. Skin patches that contain medication can be used. You can adjust your dosage to achieve adequate pain control. Rarely is it necessary at this stage to use intravenous morphine. But when needed, you can take it in the form of a controlled-dosage IV drip or even a miniature electronic injection pump through a catheter placed just under the skin. The major analgesic narcotics *will* relieve your pain if they are given in adequate dosage.

When one of my patients is not receiving acceptable pain relief from those drugs just mentioned, I check him into the hospital for treatment with an IV morphine drip. An adequate dose of this drug always relieves pain. Don't be afraid to request similar treatment if you feel you need it. Your doctor can then work with you to adjust your medication accordingly, usually switching to an oral medication plan, a skin patch, or a subcutaneous infusion.

You might worry about becoming addicted to the morphine you require for pain relief. Your anxiety is groundless. Research and clinical experience have proven that morphine taken to relieve pain rarely produces addiction.

This may seem counterintuitive because it is well established that morphine can be highly addictive among drug abusers, who take it for the euphoria it brings. Morphine addicts quickly develop a tolerance for the drug — a hallmark of addiction — and need increasing dosages to produce the same psychological effect. They also suffer physical withdrawal symptoms when deprived of the drug. These negative side effects seldom occur among cancer patients receiving analgesic morphine, however. You might experience an early but limited tolerance in which the dosage needed for pain relief increases. But this soon levels off and you do not require ever-increasing amounts. The mental clouding associated with a drug abuser's high is not a serious problem when narcotics are used as analgesics. However, withdrawal symptoms can occur if you abruptly stop the medication after having been on it for some time. If your need for pain medication decreases due to relief from a treatment such as radiation or orchiectomy, work with your doctor at gradually decreasing the dose.

Constipation might be a side effect of morphine or other opi-

Table 4. Medications for Pain

Nonnarcotic	Narcotic
Tylenol	Codeine
Nonsteroidal Anti-Inflammatory	Oxycodone
Drugs (NSAIDs)	Morphine (oral subcutaneous
Ibuprofen	or intravenous)
Naprosyn	Dilaudid
Aspirin	
Trilisate	
Steroids	

ates because narcotic analgesics slow bowel action (peristalsis). If you receive narcotic analgesics on a regular basis, drink as much fluid as possible and use stool softeners and possibly laxatives to promote intestinal motion.

Remember, you do not have to suffer in silence.

Palliative External-Beam Radiation

Radiation therapy is an effective treatment to control localized pain. Unlike the radiation administered during early prostate cancer, which has a curative goal, this treatment only relieves symptoms.

Almost as important as relieving pain, radiation of metastases can also slow bone degradation, particularly at critical weight-bearing sites such as the spine, hips, and upper legs. Though cancer cells are more vulnerable to radiation than other tissue, healthy bone marrow is also destroyed by radiation, so it is not worthwhile to request radiation as a prophylactic (preventive) measure in an attempt to delay the development of metastases. Also, bone marrow produces blood cells that you need in order to survive. Therefore, your doctor should work closely with a radiation oncologist if you choose palliative radiation therapy.

Generally, the benefits of radiation far outweigh the risks. A short course of localized radiation therapy delivered directly to the metastatic site almost always brings relief from pain within a week or two. And this relief often lasts for months or years. As in curative radiation therapy, imaging techniques can be used to precisely target the radiation beam at the metastatic site that is producing pain. During this process, your physician should strive for appropriate timing of radiation treatment.

Remember, delivering radiation too early is of uncertain value and can needlessly damage your bone marrow. A basic principle of radiation therapy is that any area of the body can receive only a given amount of radiation. This amount is measured in rads or centi-Grays, a unit of radiation energy absorbed by a given weight of tissue. Exceeding that limit will compromise your normal tissue (including bone marrow), which often will not regenerate.

The radiation of bone over time causes the total reserve of bone marrow, and thus the renewal capacity of your blood, to be compromised. A low blood count can lead to debilitation, increased risk of infection, and the need for blood transfusions. Judicious planning of palliative radiation therapy will usually prevent this negative spiral.

Your team of treating physicians must continually make judgment calls, keeping in mind your overall status. This difficult balancing act is smoother if there is good communication between you and your doctors.

The primary purpose of palliative radiation therapy is to *alleviate pain,* not to slow the growth of the cancer. When pointing to a metastatic site on a patient's bone scan, I often say, "This is one of several potential trouble spots. We will treat it if and when it begins to bother you."

Concerned that untreated bone metastases will send out more malignant seeds that will spread the cancer, you may wish to have all your known metastatic sites treated to prevent this seeding. However, cancer metastasizes in this manner only on rare occasions. The bone metastases that appear progressively in your radiographic images throughout the course of the advanced disease were probably "seeded" from your primary tumor years earlier. Once you understand this process, you'll be more comfortable with the concept of palliative radiation therapy.

Radiopharmaceuticals

We discussed the principle of treating a systemic disease by systemic means. Palliative external beam radiation, however, is localized therapy, aimed at individual metastatic sites. Its systemic equivalent is what we call radiopharmaceutical therapy.

Your doctor might suggest using a radioactive isotope such as strontium-89, which is similar to the element calcium found in your bones and is readily absorbed in areas of new bone formation. Since those areas of bone damage caused by prostate cancer metastases are the most active sites of new bone formation in your body, they will absorb the highest proportion of a radiopharmaceutical such as strontium-89. And in so doing, your metastatic sites will receive the greatest dosage of radiation from the pharmaceutical isotope.

Strontium-89, known by the brand name Metastron, has been available for a number of years. It is very effective in relieving bone pain. As an outpatient, you receive Metastron as an injection. Although there is a slight chance that you'll experience an increase in pain in the first week or so after your treatment, the process is extremely easy and straightforward. Because a proportion of the pharmaceutical is excreted in your urine, your doctor will provide a means of collecting this urine so that the radioisotope can be disposed of safely.

Some of the strontium-89 is quickly absorbed by the bony metastases. The isotope then begins to irradiate the tumor cells. If the treatment works, you'll feel significant pain relief in two to three weeks. Researchers have not yet determined whether radiopharmaceuticals slow the growth of metastases.

The radiation dose these pharmaceuticals deliver is relatively low, and most of the radiation leaves the body within hours after the injection.

Half of the strontium-89 that remains in the body disappears completely in fifty-one days. Within two to three months, you'll have excreted most of the isotope or it will have become inactivated. Pain relief can be significant during these three months. And when one dosage of strontium-89 is no longer effective, you may safely receive another dosage to continue to control your metastatic pain. After multiple injections, however, strontium-89 will degrade your bone marrow. But this risk is far outweighed by the potential important pain relieving benefits. In general, if your first injection did not work within two months, subsequent injections are not likely to help.

Other radiopharmaceuticals, including rhenium-186 and samarium-153, are being tested and may be approved in the near future for therapeutic use by the Food and Drug Administration.

If you have painful prostate cancer bone metastases, you're probably a good candidate for radiopharmaceuticals. Discuss the appropriate time to use this treatment with your doctor. What about the side effects? In the more advanced stage of the disease, side effects such as bone marrow compromise are less important on your risk-benefit curve than the significant pain relief radiopharmaceuticals can bring you.

The Risk of Fracture

Bone fractures can also cause metastatic pain. If bone becomes weakened by either blastic overgrowth or, more commonly, lytic destruction, it can break. Thankfully, bone fractures are unusual in the case of prostate cancer. Major fractures might be preceded by painful smaller breaks. In either case, this pain can be intense, and the bone trauma itself can cause you serious complications. The risk of fracture typically can be ascertained by an X-ray of the bone in question.

The greater concern regarding fracture is in your weight-bearing bones, which might have metastases. If sharp pain suddenly flares up in a particular spot, ask your doctor if you need X-rays to check for a fracture. Your primary physician might also consult closely with orthopedic specialists, as I do, in order to intervene before an important structural bone suffers fracture.

Sometimes an orthopedist or radiologist will spot a problem well before it is critical. "This is a bone I'm worried about," the consulting physician might say, pointing to an X-ray plate.

In such a case, your doctor might recommend surgical intervention — the insertion of a light metal reinforcement rod or pin to strengthen the bone. The decision to do this is complex, and you should avoid surgery that is unnecessary. However, the fracture of an important weight-bearing bone such as a femur, hip bone, or lumbar vertebra is a devastating setback, causing immobility and the possibility of becoming bedridden. If your doctors can help prevent this negative turn of events through a surgical procedure and it otherwise makes sense for you, it should be done.

From a preventive standpoint, activity is important for strong bones and muscles. You should keep up non-traumatic exercise such as walking and swimming. Dietary calcium supplements and vitamin D are of uncertain benefit in preventing fracture.

Fortunately, once again, prostate cancer metastases cause relatively more blastic (overgrowth) than destructive (lytic) bone change, compared to other malignancies such as metastatic breast cancer.

Case Histories: Palliative Radiation and Radiopharmaceutical Therapies

Anthony T. is a 68-year-old recently retired textile worker from northern New Hampshire, who underwent a radical prostatectomy for prostate cancer fifteen years ago. In 1988, although Anthony felt perfectly well, his doctor recommended the new

PSA test. Not wanting to think about recurrent prostate cancer, Anthony avoided taking the test then, but finally did so in 1990. He was deeply troubled by the results: a PSA level 15.0 ng/ml. This was strongly suggestive of metastatic prostate cancer because his prostate had been surgically removed fifteen years earlier. The next PSA in July 1991, revealed a clearly rising trend: 32.0 ng/ml.

Although Anthony's bone scan and CT scan were normal, he and his doctor decided to start hormonal treatment. Anthony underwent an orchiectomy in late 1991. His PSA decreased to 1.6 ng/ml by January 1992.

Over the next few years, Anthony's PSA began to climb. By January 1995 his PSA had reached 30.0 ng/ml and his bone scan showed metastases in the spine and one femur. Then a metastatic site showed up in his left shoulder. Anthony's team of physicians treated him with a variety of other hormonal and antiandrogen medications. Anthony also received two courses of palliative external-beam radiation. The first radiation was to his lower back, followed a month later by a treatment of his left shoulder. This palliative radiation brought very quick, and long-lasting, pain relief.

At that point, Anthony's doctor suggested that he consult with me. When he came to my clinic, Anthony stated that he had lost ten pounds over the past six months and was taking nonsteroidal analgesics, as well as the opiate MS Contin at a dosage of 30 milligrams twice a day. But his serious back pain persisted. He needed about four additional narcotic-analgesic tablets a day to withstand this breakthrough pain.

I ordered a new bone scan, which revealed many new metastatic sites on his lower spine and pelvic bones. When I discussed treatment options with Anthony, he was not interested in chemotherapy or any experimental protocols. "I just want to live out my time as comfortably as I can," he said.

I recommended the radiopharmaceutical strontium, which was simple to take and effective. Within two weeks of Anthony's first strontium injection, he was free of pain. His appetite improved and he managed to gain weight.

Today Anthony is on his third course of injected strontium pharmaceutical and is doing very well.

Neurological Impairment

A problem that is sometimes associated with bone metastases is neurological impairment, or nerve damage. This occurs when tumor tissue compresses nerves (typically the nerves in the spinal column). A combination of bone damage might destabilize one or more vertebrae, particularly in your mid (thoracic) or lower (lumbar) region, causing compression of the spinal cord and its important ganglia. The ganglia descend through channels in the bony pelvis to your legs. A common symptom of neurological impairment is persistent back pain, so you should be alert to this warning.

If left untreated, neurological impairment might cause weakness in your feet or legs or a rapid onset of urinary or rectal incontinence. Neurological impairment in other areas of the spinal column can cause strange sensations. You might suffer a disturbing loss of positional sense: suddenly you will not feel the placement of your legs and feet. Nerve impairment also can cause abnormal sensations of heat or cold.

As with any neurological disorder, these symptoms can form complex and confusing combinations. *Any* unusual neurological symptom, including weakness in one of your limbs or sensory anomalies, such as numbness or tingling, should be reported to your physician immediately.

Modern MRI scanning equipment provides excellent images of the spinal column and its network of nerves. If neurological impairment due to bone change or the pressure of metastatic tumors is detected on the scan, your doctor has a range of treatment options available, including localized external-beam radiation and medical therapies such as steroids. Sometimes surgery is needed.

The Last Stages of Metastatic Prostate Cancer

I do not intend to dwell morosely on the last phases of metastatic prostate cancer. Everyone reading this book — whether or not you are ill — understands that death is inevitable. However, I promised at the outset to be both frank and compassionate in discussing the impact of this disease on you and your family. Moreover, a review of the popular literature on prostate cancer shows that most writers, including my fellow physicians, avoid discussing terminal prostate cancer. This may only add to your anxiety. You and your family want to know as much as possible about the final phase of the disease in order to prepare yourselves emotionally for the inevitable. Therefore, I will share the knowledge that I have gained in treating men who eventually died of the disease.

Prostate cancer does not usually cause death by encroaching on a vital organ or system, as in some other cancers. Instead, men eventually succumb to what we call the total tumor burden. This process varies among individuals, but usually follows a predictable pattern.

After periods of remission, the man slips into a progressive decline. Whatever palliative treatment had previously succeeded in slowing the progress of the cancer is no longer effective.

Sometimes there will be an increase in the pain from bone metastases. But this pain can still be managed with analgesic narcotics, principally intravenous morphine. However, it is often necessary to increase the dosage of medications during this period.

Bone metastases also can interfere with the man's reserves of bone marrow, necessitating transfusions to replace the blood no longer produced by the marrow. During this period, there may be day-to-day fluctuations in the man's sense of well-being: he may have days of renewed vigor and days of fatigue and listlessness. Ultimately the man's energy is sapped to the point that he becomes bedridden.

Prostate cancer patients do not generally experience the severe emaciation that is often associated with terminal cancer. But the man's appetite will often fluctuate before major debilitation occurs. If you reach this stage, you may lose interest in food, and eating the traditional three meals a day may not be appealing. I advise you to find food you like — be it the healthiest granola bar or a McDonald's cheeseburger — and eat small portions periodically throughout the day. If a glass of wine at noon or sundown makes your food more palatable, all the better. You might wish to augment these small meals with commercially available dietary supplements such as Ensure. But I have found that most patients arrive at a balance of food they enjoy and can tolerate easily. If you eat less on some days or miss occasional meals, this does not make the cancer worse and certainly does not mean that you are losing the battle.

The tumor burden can compromise the immune system, and infections such as pneumonia become life threatening. Unfortunately, bone marrow impingement compromises blood-clotting ability, and bleeding may rarely occur. The opposite also can occur: blood clots. Each person has a different course, and in any individual the course may vary. My best advice is what I tell all my patients at this stage: "Take it one day at a time." You will have good days and bad days. You might well experience periods during which you have renewed energy; you'll feel well enough to go out for dinner, take a walk, or go to a movie.

In the man's last months, he can usually be treated comfortably at home. His caregivers, either family or professional, can manage even an intravenous drip for the administration of fluids or pain medications. Therefore, about 90 percent of advanced prostate cancer patients die at home. Most people want to be at home, and this is certainly feasible if desirable.

This situation presents a problem if you have an elderly or

infirm wife who is not able to provide an adequate level of care. Grown children are often widely dispersed, so they are not able to act as caregivers. If this situation exists, you and your family should consult with your physician and the clinical social workers responsible for your case.

Hospice care has become quite sophisticated in America. A man in the final phase of metastatic prostate cancer may usually receive all the professional care he requires in a hospice setting, which is often less stressful on him and his family than a general hospital. The man's final days are usually marked by periods of sleep and drowsy wakefulness.

12

Metastatic Prostate Cancer III: Systemic and Experimental Treatment of the Cancer

Management Strategies Beyond Hormonal Therapy

There is a principle underlying every treatment for metastatic prostate cancer that is deceptively simple: try to find a therapy that kills the cancer cells or slows their growth throughout the body. Medicine has been only modestly successful in meeting this goal. This can also be said for other malignancies, including breast and colorectal cancer.

Metastatic prostate cancer is a systemic (bodywide) disease, not a local disease. Therefore, any therapy that slows your disease must be systemic in its approach. It is this principle that underlies hormonal therapy. And, as we have seen, this approach usually produces a significant remission of disease which prolongs your life and improves your quality of life.

Your physician may supplement the strategy of systemic treatment with specific tactics of local treatment. This might include local palliative radiation therapy to alleviate metastatic pain or metastatic impairment of your spinal cord and its branches. If called for, surgical intervention repairs or prevents structural bone damage.

Your realistic goal during this combined treatment is similar to that of hormonal ablation therapy: maintain a good quality of life for as long as possible.

Second-Line Hormonal Therapy

Here are some questions you should ask if you are reaching the effective end of conventional hormonal therapy.

What happens when hormonal therapy finally fails?

As I described earlier, when initial hormonal therapy fails, you have some cancer cells that can grow in low concentrations of male hormone. So you should consider treatments that are still hormonal in nature after your remission comes to an end.

How will I know my remission is over?

A rising PSA trend is the most obvious sign that remission has ended and the disease is progressing.

What should I do then?

The first thing to do if you have been taking flutamide (Eulexin) or bicalutamide (Casodex) is stop taking these drugs. These antiandrogens prevent hormonally sensitive prostate cells from interacting with male hormones. Once combined hormonal deprivation and antiandrogen therapy is no longer effective because of the proliferation of hormone refractory tumor cells, you no longer need flutamide or bicalutamide. And we now know that at this stage of disease flutamide or bicalutamide can actually stimulate the growth of some of the prostate cancer cells.

Will this help slow the growth of the cancer?

Stopping flutamide or bicalutamide, but continuing the LH-RH analog component results in a remission in about one third of advanced prostate cancer patients. If you've had an orchiectomy, this means simply stopping the pills. The remission usually lasts for months, but rarely years.

Why shouldn't I also stop LH-RH agonist therapy?

Because you probably have a small surviving reserve of hormonally sensitive cells within the cancer that must be suppressed through androgen deprivation. In theory, unless you continue to deprive these cells of male hormones, they might grow more vigorously.

What other treatments can help me now?

First, you should realize that if you have undergone an orchiectomy, using leuprolide (Lupron) or gosereline (Zoladex) will not help. Moreover, if you have been using an LH-RH analog, an orchiectomy will not likely be of benefit, although you might choose to have the surgery to avoid the monthly injections.

After a trial of stopping either flutamide or bicalutamide, it may be worthwhile to try the other drug in its place. This may generate a remission. If you had been on Eulexin before, starting Casodex (usually at 150 mg/day) may work. Conversely, trying Eulexin after stopping Casodex may help. If this has failed, you can turn to another group of drugs, including ketoconazole, that interferes with the production of hormones from your adrenal glands. Remember, even with hormonal therapy your adrenal glands may produce enough androgen to help surviving hormonally sensitive malignant cells grow. So ask your doctor about a course of ketoconazole (also called Nizoral) or a drug called aminoglutethimide, which can very quickly suppress the production of male hormones in your adrenal glands and in so doing bring a remission in your cancer.[1]

Are these drugs safe?

Ketoconazole rarely causes major side effects at normal doses, but might have some at higher doses. You might suffer diarrhea, nausea, or indigestion, but this can be managed with medication. Some men develop fatigue. In some cases, these side effects make use of the drug prohibitive. Ketoconazole should not be taken with meals because it won't be absorbed from your gastrointestinal tract. Aminoglutethimide is tolerable, but it may cause a rash that takes a few days to disappear. Both of these drugs are frequently used together with low doses of steroids.

What if my PSA continues to rise?

If your PSA continues to rise after ketoconazole or aminoglutethimide therapy, this is an indication that a major proportion of the malignant cell mass is now hormonally insensitive (refractory).

Chemotherapy

What is chemotherapy?

Chemotherapy involves toxic compounds, most of which are derived from substances found in nature. If hormonal therapy deprives prostate cancer cells of the androgen "food" they need, chemotherapy actually poisons some of these cells.

Will chemotherapy help me?

You should ask your doctor's opinion. He might recommend it. In general, I reserve the use of chemotherapy for those patients who have symptoms from their cancer. A medical oncologist would normally administer and supervise this treatment.

But you should also honestly assess how you and your doctor view treatment for metastatic prostate cancer. First, you have to be flexible. Problems can wax and wane; that is, problem areas change, new metastases might appear, and older metastatic sites might suddenly flare up or present a risk of structural bone or nerve damage.

If you respond to chemotherapy, there is often an alleviation of the severity and duration of pain or other symptoms, as well as an improvement in your overall vigor and psychological state.

Does palliative chemotherapy really do me any good?

Palliative treatment is meant to relieve your symptoms. But it's logical to assume that any form of treatment that slows or dampens metastatic tumor growth will add time to your life. In oncology, the life-prolonging aspect of palliative therapy is controversial. Effective palliation could add weeks and months — and in a few cases, years — to the lives of advanced prostate cancer patients. Moreover, the quality of your life during this survival period is almost always enhanced.

So, in the spirit of treating advanced disease aggressively, your doctor may recommend chemotherapy. This may seem illogical because I have already noted that chemotherapy is only a modestly effective treatment in prostate cancer. However, if you consider chemotherapy as only one of several palliative treatments available, its use makes more sense.

Can it cure my prostate cancer?

With the drugs we currently have available, chemotherapy cannot cure prostate cancer. In fact, the cure rate for chemotherapy in other forms of metastatic cancer is also not very good.[2]

The goal of chemotherapy for prostate cancer patients is to improve your quality of life. And this therapy can sometimes bring remission.

Is the treatment safe?

The chemotherapy drugs often used for advanced prostate cancer are not as toxic as those used in treating other malignancies. My basic philosophy regarding chemotherapy is to maximize the benefits of the treatment while minimizing the negative side effects.

What type of chemotherapy should I ask for?

The types of chemotherapy that I currently use most often include a pill called estramustine (Emcyt). I use this in combination with other drugs, including vinblastine, Etoposide, or Taxol. These three drugs are given intravenously, but Etoposide can also be given as a pill.

What about side effects?

The side effects of these combinations are usually less severe than with other forms of chemotherapy. In fact, you'll probably be able to function at near-normal levels during this therapy. You'll experience a little nausea and some hair loss. But overall, the benefits of this chemotherapy tend to outweigh the risk of the generally tolerable side effects.

Are there other chemotherapy drugs for prostate cancer?

These combinations of medications are but a few of the types of chemotherapy used. Other regimens can also be effective. If chemotherapy is an option, it is up to you and your physician to work closely together to find the right combination.

How long should I continue chemotherapy?

If chemotherapy seems to relieve pain and improve your

strength, and you are tolerating the side effects, continue the treatment indefinitely. However, if there is no marked improvement, as is the case for many patients, discontinue chemotherapy.[3]

Case History: Second-line Hormonal Therapy and Chemotherapy

Jack R., 78, was diagnosed with prostate cancer in 1991. He'd suffered symptoms of an enlarged prostate for several years and was under the active scrutiny of a urologist due to mild to moderate urinary problems. When Jack did not respond to standard medications, his urologist ordered a PSA assay. At that time the test was just beginning to be used. Jack's PSA was elevated: 30.0 ng/ml. A sextant biopsy revealed prostate cancer in three of the six cores. The grade of Jack's tumor was $3 + 4 = 7$ on the Gleason score.

Given his age and other medical problems, Jack opted for radiation therapy. After a standard course, however, his PSA showed a steadily rising trend, evidence of metastatic disease that had obviously spread before the radiation therapy. Several months later, Jack's bone scan was positive and his PSA was rising fast, into the 150 ng/ml range.

Jack began standard hormonal treatment with an LH-RH analog. After several months, however, he chose to undergo an orchiectomy because it was more convenient. Jack's PSA dropped dramatically, and his cancer went into remission for three years.

However, the cancer recurred, and Jack began to suffer typical symptoms of general aching. His physician referred him to me. A bone scan revealed widespread metastatic involvement of Jack's leg bones, ribs, and parts of his skull. I noticed that he had swelling around his left eye. I immediately ordered an MRI, which, as I suspected, showed metastatic sites in the bones around that eye.

Because this was a crisis, I asked my radiation oncology colleagues if Jack could begin palliative radiation that afternoon.

They took him to the center for his first course of spot radiation that evening.

Since Jack had undergone orchiectomy, I thought it might be worthwhile to start a course of ketoconazole, in the hope that some of the cells in the tumor might respond. Within weeks, Jack responded to this second line of hormonal therapy and also the radiation. His aches disappeared and his eye returned to normal. Jack's PSA level had risen to 700 ng/ml, but with the medication it dropped to 50 ng/ml. For the next six months, while on ketoconazole, Jack had no symptoms and required no pain medications. This was a happy, productive period for him, during which he took several pleasant trips with his grandchildren.

By the seventh month, however, Jack's aches had returned and his PSA had risen back over 100 ng/ml. It was clear that the hormonally refractive cells of his cancer were reasserting themselves. I suggested a course of chemotherapy. Neither of us expected a dramatic remission, but we were both hopeful of a good palliative effect. Jack began chemotherapy using a combination of two drugs, estramustine (Emcyt) and vinblastine (Velban). He tolerated this chemotherapy very well, with only slight nausea. More importantly, Jack's pain began to improve markedly after three weeks.

Experimental Treatments

Cancer in general, and prostate cancer in particular, is a complex and often unpredictable disease. Accordingly, the medical and scientific communities and pharmaceutical industry are constantly seeking new forms of effective treatment. In the ongoing process of this search, a number of promising therapies periodically arise, some proving to be effective while others are less so than originally hoped.

Why should I take an unproven experimental treatment?

Experimental treatments play a critical role in medicine and can be especially important in cancer therapy. Any new treatment must first be clinically tested in trial protocols in order to carefully assess their benefits and side effects. Although this might seem to you like a frustrating trial-and-error process, effective new prostate cancer treatments will undoubtedly arise from experimental protocols under way. Engaging in such trials may help you and will definitely help others in the future.

New Drugs: Suramin

The drug suramin was considered one of the promising experimental therapies when it began to be used to treat metastatic prostate cancer about ten years ago. Suramin was originally developed to treat African sleeping sickness, a form of encephalitis caused by an insect-borne parasite. But researchers discovered the drug also had a profound effect on cellular replication.[4]

Clinical trials of suramin proved that the drug had multiple effects, including suppressing the adrenal glands. It has since been used for experimental prostate cancer therapy.

Will suramin help me?

Suramin is currently being tested in experimental therapy protocols. Although there are indications that the drug relieves pain and/or reduces the PSA in some patients, its true benefits are not yet established.

When suramin was first used, its side effects were almost prohibitive. Today the doses have been modified, and most people tolerate suramin without problems. If you think you are a candidate for suramin treatment, you may wish to discuss your entry into clinical trials with your doctor.

New Drugs: Chemotherapy

New drugs that kill cancer cells (called cytotoxic drugs) are constantly being evaluated. Such agents that are currently being tested in prostate cancer are havelbine, high-dose cyclophosphamide, and liposome-encapsulated dexorobin or adriamycin.

New Drugs: Therapies Targeting Tumor Metastasis

What other new treatments might be available in the future?

One interesting experimental treatment approach is called antiangiogenesis therapy. Several years ago, Judah Folkman, a pioneering surgeon at Harvard Medical School, recognized that tumors needed an enhanced blood supply (neovasculature) to fulfill their malignant growth potential. Neovasculature begins with the tiny extension of capillaries into the growing malignant tumor mass, whether a primary tumor, such as an organ-confined prostate cancer, or its metastases.

Researchers are developing drugs to block the secretions that stimulate neovasculature in tumors. If this is successful, prostate tumors and many other cancers will be deprived of the blood supply they need for uncontrolled malignant growth. Researchers have identified drugs that appear to stymie neovasculature development in some malignant tissues.[5] These are currently undergoing clinical trials.

Another promising approach is to interfere with a tumor's ability to invade tissue. This process of invasion is dependent on enzymes or proteins that are produced by the tumor itself or even by the normal tissue, which has been stimulated by the tumor. Interfering with these enzymes may suppress the invasive ability of a tumor. One such group of enzymes, metalloproteinases, are critical to this process. Drugs that inhibit these enzymes are now in clinical trial for prostate cancer.

When tumor cells metastasize, the cells must attach to something for them to take root and grow. Interfering with this attachment process might prevent or delay the development of prostate cancer. Modified citrus pectin, a naturally occurring protein/sugar complex, has been shown to prevent metastasis in animal models and will soon be tested in clinical trials.

New Treatments: Genetics and Gene Therapy

What other experimental treatments show promise?

As we learn more about the genetic changes that occur during the development of prostate cancer, we will better understand which genes need to be "fixed" or which biochemical pathway that these genes control needs to be repaired. Drug screening for the small molecules that target specific genes is an active enterprise now, which will likely grow as new target genes are discovered. It is hoped that basic scientific information regarding altered genes will lead to development of new drugs and to strategies to repair genes. This approach is called gene therapy. It is too early to know when the benefits of this approach will be realized.

The Immune System and Immunotherapy

Can my immune system be strengthened to fight prostate cancer?

The concept behind this experimental therapeutic approach is to mobilize your body's own defenses, the immune system, against cancer.

Your immune system uses a variety of components to identify and defend against foreign material in your body. We are constantly mustering an immunological response to a host of outside agents, ranging from microbes all the way to transplanted organs. Unfortunately, our immune system responds weakly to malignant tissue and generally does not recognize a primary tumor or its metastases as alien substances. This is because the cells of the tumor contain the genetic information unique to each of us.

If, however, your immune system could be altered so that its defensive components recognize malignant tissue as alien and attack it, you would gain a powerful new weapon to fight cancer. One of the major theoretical advantages of this approach would be that only tumor cells, not your normal tissue, would be targeted and attacked by the immune system. This is the goal of immunotherapy.

The potential vulnerability of cancer cells to suppression by your own immune system was discovered when metastatic tumors were seen to be suppressed in patients with rampant infections. The immune system produces substances called cytokines, complex proteins normally secreted in response to a variety of normal stimuli. These cytokines include interferon and interleukin-2, which is secreted by the white blood cells (lymphocytes) we call T cells.[6]

Can I benefit from immunotherapy?

The benefits of immunotherapy for prostate cancer have not yet been established. Immunotherapy most likely will not produce a single magic cure for prostate cancer. Your immune system is extremely complex, and much still needs to be learned about it. But progress is being made through the enrollment of patients who volunteer for experimental treatment protocols.

Immunotherapy promises to eventually provide a powerful tool that can perhaps be combined with other treatments to produce significant remissions of metastatic prostate cancer during the hormone refractory phase of the disease. Ask your doctor if you're a good candidate for such an approach.

New Treatments: Vaccines

What about vaccines against prostate cancer?

Vaccines stimulate the immune system. The strategy behind traditional vaccines has usually been to activate the immune system to fight foreign proteins, such as those in a virus. The polio vaccine was developed to do this. Cancer vaccines are far more complex because your body's immune system does not recognize cancer as a foreign cell or tissue. Thus, vaccines for cancer involve reteaching or fooling your immune system that a cancer cell is foreign. Such strategies are under development in prostate cancer using a variety of prostate-specific proteins such as PSA and prostate-specific membrane antigen, PSM.

Combining Gene Therapy with Immunotherapy

Are other approaches being developed that will aid the the immune system?

An innovative approach to immunotherapy was developed by my Dana-Farber colleague, Glenn Dranoff, while working with Richard Mulligan of Massachusetts Institute of Technology.

Dranoff's approach is to genetically alter cancer cells to make them vulnerable to the immune system. To do this, cancer cells are first grown in a laboratory dish; then, by genetic engineering, a gene called granulocyte-macrophage colony stimulating factor (GMCSF) is introduced into the cancer cells. The genetically altered cells are then irradiated to prevent their further reproduction. Finally, the cells are introduced into laboratory mice. The cells act as a vaccine or a stimulant of the immune system, affecting the growth of tumor cells in the rodent. The "vaccination" stimulated the immune system to seek out and destroy malignant cells.

This type of immunotherapy is now being tested with some success in patients with kidney cancer. It is hoped that this approach will eventually prove beneficial in treating metastatic prostate cancer. Trial protocols of this promising immunotherapy approach began in 1996.

Ask your doctor if you are a good candidate for this promising experimental treatment. Physicians and investigators recognize that progress is made through clinical trials; participating in a clinical trial protocol might be beneficial to you. And your involvement will certainly help others. Further, most men I have worked with in clinical trials appreciate the chance to receive the new — but unproven — therapy before it is approved for wider use.

Support for Research into Experimental Treatment

The heightened public awareness of prostate cancer has rejuvenated clinical research in the field. Michael Milken, an advanced prostate cancer patient, has helped stimulate this upsurge in research by privately funding studies and clinical trials across the country. And as the awareness of the incidence of the disease increases — as it surely will, given the increased use of the PSA assay — more support for research, public and private, will undoubtedly be forthcoming.

Quackery and Questionable Treatment

Are there any quacks or charlatans in the field?
A truly unfortunate aspect of treating cancer patients is the presence of individuals who are ready to exploit vulnerable people. You should keep this sad fact in mind as you consider experimental treatments.

We need only consider the upsurge of laetrile clinics across the United States–Mexico border in the 1960s (established to avoid United States health codes) to understand the negative impact of exploitation on cancer patients and their families. Quackery potentially deprives you of proper treatment and also leads to unrealistic expectations and financial loss.

Should I avoid all unproven treatments?
No. I occasionally encounter questionable therapeutic claims regarding treatment of prostate cancer. However, I always try to keep an open mind, recognizing that tomorrow's cure might well have been today's unorthodox experimental therapy.

However, you must balance this optimistic view with a cold eye toward outright fraud and exploitation. If you hear of a "miracle" cure (generally very expensive) that is offered only in some obscure foreign clinic, be very skeptical.

What are these questionable treatments?

One is the use of dried shark cartilage, which is being touted as a cancer treatment. Although there is evidence that supports that it has antiangiogenic properties, its proponents state that ingesting a substantial amount of shark cartilage — about 100 grams a day — will bring remission in metastatic prostate cancer. The logic behind this approach is that many species of sharks do not seem to develop malignant tumors, supposedly because they possess a potent, naturally occurring antiangiogenic substance. Proponents further state this substance can be metabolized by human beings with beneficial effect.

There is currently no evidence that shark cartilage has any benefit in treating or preventing cancer. But scientific investigation of shark cartilage is under way.

Another claim that unreasonably raises hope among prostate cancer patients is that the macrobiotic diet will bring remission in metastatic disease. This diet came into vogue in America during the 1960s, when it was seen by many young people as a panacea for spiritual and physical health. The diet is based on whole grains and is practically devoid of animal protein and saturated fats. There is no reliable scientific evidence that this radical dietary regimen has any beneficial effect whatsoever on the course of prostate cancer.

What about megavitamin therapy?

Similar claims of remarkable therapeutic efficacity have been made for megadoses of certain vitamins, notably the antioxidants, including vitamins C, E, and A. Although antioxidant vitamins probably play some role in the dietary prevention of cancer, there is no evidence that greatly increasing vitamin intake to extraordinary levels plays any beneficial role at all in the remission of metastatic prostate cancer.

How can I avoid being tricked?

First, talk with your doctor before taking any treatments. And bear in mind that one of the common factors among these questionable alternative therapies is the overstated claims of benefit.

Lacking the documentation of careful clinical trials, the proponents of these treatments often claim dramatic or significant success for the product or process they favor. And the motives of some of these advocates are clearly questionable. Although not virtually snake oil, some of these miracle cures are close to it.

Who can I trust?

Use your common sense when considering these unorthodox treatment approaches. Try to keep an open mind, but don't fall for high-pressure sales pitches. Normally I tell my patients: "Let me know what you're doing so I can learn with you." Thus far, however, I have not been impressed by these miracle cures.

Some unconventional approaches are relatively benign, and I recognize that the hope of remission they represent can be an essential ingredient in your emotional well-being.

I encountered a troubling practice with a literary critic who came to me with advanced metastatic disease. When our palliative therapy ultimately failed to produce a significant remission, he returned to New York, where he underwent a form of questionable treatment. It consisted of a prolonged but utterly useless series of coffee enemas which supposedly had great therapeutic potential.

Common sense is a valuable tool when you are weighing the potential benefit of an unorthodox or highly unusual form of therapy. If the treatment has been available for several years but no major medical institution or pharmaceutical company has shown interest in it, you should be skeptical of its usefulness.

13

Where to Turn for Help

Psychosocial Support

If you have been diagnosed with advanced metastatic prostate cancer, I'm sure you have gone through emotional turmoil, with periods of anxious denial, hopelessness, loneliness, and perhaps depression. But you and your family do not have to shoulder this heavy burden alone.

There are many forms of psychosocial support available to you. Your hospital probably has psychiatric or oncology clinic nurse specialists, as well as clinical social workers who have been specifically trained to work with people in your situation. Clergy and layperson counselors from your church or synagogue are also trained in helping patients and their families during this difficult period. And you may find private psychologists and psychiatrists helpful for individual or family counseling.

As you enter this frightening period of your life, you can learn from those who have been here before you.

Point One: Communicate your feelings. Even though it may be difficult for you to talk about the impact your disease has had on your life, the lack of discussion of painful issues within families can become destructive. From my experience in working with people in your position, I've learned that it is important to talk, to express your emotions, deal with the issues, and involve your family and close friends. And don't hesitate to seek advice and consultation from social workers and psychiatrists. The team approach — you, your family and friends, and your professional supporters — is essential.

At each phase of the disease, different goals and priorities emerge. You'll be better able to deal with the last phases of the disease when you know all reasonable treatment measures have been exhausted, and you will have gained confidence that metastatic pain is manageable.

Point Two: Even the strongest individual often becomes depressed as the disease advances. If you are hit with significant depression, seek help from a psychiatrist or clinical psychologist. Your clergy can refer you to professionals who are trained to treat this type of depression. Treatment can be in the form of joint counseling with you and your family or other psychotherapy administered in combination with antidepressant medications.

Your family members should be alert to the signs of depression, both in you and among themselves. The judicious use of antidepressant medications may make you feel better, function more efficiently, and allow you to determine your own priorities at this stage of your life.

Point Three: Put the practical aspects of your life in order early in the process so you don't feel pressured to make snap decisions later on. You will be more comfortable if you take part in the necessary legal and financial arrangements connected with the end of your life. These include updating your will and arranging power of attorney to handle your affairs should you become incapacitated. If your family normally consults a certified public accountant for your tax and financial affairs, you should discuss the appropriate procedures with your accountant at this time. You may also want to draw up a living will, which many states require, if you do not wish to have extraordinary resuscitation measures taken by health care providers. Your attorney should be able to arrange this in a tactful manner.

Point Four: During periods when you are feeling well, indulge yourself in a vacation or other luxury that you have always dreamed of but never enjoyed. Now is the time to see Paris in the spring, make a pilgrimage to Rome, or visit Israel. This time in your life does not have to become an endless preoccupation with your own mortality.

A gift to yourself may involve your children or grandchildren: seats on the 50-yard line at an NFL game or a fishing trip to the Florida Keys. The nature of the event is less important than the act of self-fulfillment it represents. Periods of remission offer the chance to relish your life with loved ones.

Point Five: Members of the clergy urge men to mend fences with estranged family members or friends during this period. You should take their advice.

Point Six: Enjoy life's small pleasures. You'll probably find heightened joy in your children and grandchildren. And you will find satisfaction in the simple pleasures most of us take for granted. Think of my patient who makes a detour each day in the park to observe the change of the seasons and the progress of the flowerbeds and trees.

Some men seek out their childhood homes and boyhood friends, not to undergo an emotionally wrenching catharsis but simply to renew pleasant memories.

A note to family members: You can be supportive during this period by driving your loved one to the places he requests, even if they seem unusual. A man in his 70s with metastatic prostate cancer undoubtedly has good reason for wanting to see a dilapidated old factory where he served his apprenticeship or to stroll a weedy baseball diamond where he was initiated into the mysteries of a catcher's mitt.

Point Seven: Savor your good memories. In the final phases of the disease there might be periods of weeks during which symptoms abate and your vigor returns. This can be a time of satisfying reflection on your achievements. You may choose to set down the events of your life in a personalized photo album, a journal, or in letters to your grandchildren; in this way you'll pass on to another generation an informal history of your family. Or you may wish to join the oral history projects sponsored by many colleges and universities in the United States so that you can personally contribute to the living record of your community.

Advice for Wives of Patients

Some men deal with stress by using different coping mechanisms than do women. Your loved one with prostate cancer may grow emotionally through the experience of coping with this serious disease. He may accept the diagnosis of cancer as a wake-up call to enjoy life, to live for the moment.

Carl H., a physician, promptly retired after being diagnosed with prostate cancer, which had metastasized to his lymph nodes. He has become an avid reader and traveler; he now has more time to enjoy these activities. Most remarkably, this change in his life has brought on a new closeness and intimacy with his wife.

Conversely, your loved one might become depressed and morose, finding it difficult to see a sense of purpose in his life. The stark, unremitting diagnosis of cancer may send him into an emotional tailspin.

The consequences of treatment often are extremely difficult to cope with. They have parallels to breast cancer therapy: after undergoing mastectomy, a woman's sexual self-image may by negatively altered. Often, her significant other helps her regain confidence in intimate relations. The low self-image your loved one feels after treatment for prostate cancer may result in sexual dysfunction, a feeling of undesirability. Only your support will make it better. Your loved one most likely will have difficulty discussing changes in sexual function. He will also no doubt have trouble discussing incontinence, which he may see as a loss of control of his body. Your first positive steps together are to acknowledge these changes and the feelings that accompany them. Providing opportunities for frank discussion allows for different approaches to satisfy both your needs.

Men are usually less verbal than women, particularly about their concerns and fears: they often deal with such issues on their own terms. Your loved one does need your support, but may seek it in different ways. He may turn to you about all his concerns or he may turn to you only about certain matters. Don't be surprised or hurt if he relies heavily on his close friends and doctor and less heavily on you. He may also turn to support groups. For your loved one, the knowledge that you are simply available is sufficient, and he will turn to you when he can.

In my experience, marriages in which the wife is not permitted to be a major part of the man's support system leads to frustration for the wife. If this happens to you, consult your health care professionals for guidance.

Another important point to keep in mind: your loved one (like many men) may be much more trusting of the medical establishment and less questioning than you are. Due to social and political changes, women have often already gained self-empowerment with regard to managing their own health. Because women hear things and respond differently than men do in consultations, women should attend as many consultations with their loved one as possible. Then both partners can better digest the information they receive.

In my years as a physician caring for men with prostate cancer, I have come to the conclusion that the only thing that matches the courage and will of the patients is the courage and commitment of their wives. Much like men, women cope with prostate cancer in different ways. If you work outside the house, you'll need to find extra time to meet the challenges, and this will add a significant amount of stress to an already trying situation. Remember that women cope with stress, turmoil, or despair in varying ways. Some turn to family; others turn to friends. Your husband's doctor should be your advocate as well. He or she should help you sort out priorities and help you make plans. Your husband's physician can also arrange for you to seek help with other health care providers.

Many support groups have sessions for the wives, which you'll find extremely useful. And make sure to set aside time for yourself.

Patient Support Groups

Many men with prostate cancer receive emotional assistance and valuable information about the disease by joining patient support and advocacy groups. Such groups are established at cancer centers and hospitals nationwide. The most active international prostate cancer patient support organization is US Too, founded in 1990.

Us Too provides information, phone support, and referrals, among other services, and a newsletter. Contact: Us Too International, Inc., 930 North York Road, Suite 50, Hinsdale, Illinois, 60521-2993; their toll-free number is 1-800-808-7866. For further information, contact Us Too on the World Wide Web at http://www.ustoo.com.

In a group, you'll share a common bond and often be able to pass on to fellow members important information about treatment options that some men would have otherwise missed.

The American Foundation for Urologic Disease also coordinates the Prostate Cancer Support Group Network (PCSGN). To obtain information on patient support groups in your community, contact PCSGN: 300 W. Pratt St., Suite 401, Baltimore, MD 21201. Their toll-free number is: (800) 828-7866 or (800) 822-5277. This network also provides free information about clinical trials and the latest advances in therapy.

Other sources of information on prostate cancer and its side effects include:

American Cancer Society: (800) 227-2345 [800-ACS-2345]
Bladder Health Council: (800) 435-2732
Man To Man, Inc./ACS: (800) 227-2345
National Cancer Institute, Information, PDQ, CANCERFAX:
    (800) 422-6237 [800-4CANCER]
Patient Advocates for Advanced Cancer Treatment (PAACT):
    (616) 453-1477

Prostate Health Council: (800) 242-2383
Help for Incontinent People: (800) 252-3337 [800-BLADDER]
Simon Foundation for Continence: (800) 237-4666
Sexual Function Health Council: (800) 242-2383
Coping, Living With Cancer (magazine): (615) 790-2400

These support groups provide one-on-one information for both you and your family members, day and night. Experienced survivors provide counseling to all seeking information, especially newly diagnosed early prostate cancer patients.

In a typical support group meeting, you will hear a lecture by a professional, often a physician treating prostate cancer, followed by questions from the audience. This assembly is usually followed by smaller "breakout" groups focusing on specialized topics. If you're a newly diagnosed man who has not yet chosen treatment options but are considering surgery or radiation, you'll find these discussions especially valuable. If you're recovering from treatment and suffer side effects, you'll gain valuable information in these smaller groups. And there are groups available for advanced-disease survivors who have their own requirements. Finally, women-only breakout groups allow wives and family members to share their experiences and counsel each other.

Perhaps most importantly, these self-help and support groups make clear to the man with prostate cancer and to his family that they are not alone in their struggle against the disease.

Computer information on prostate cancer can be obtained online by searching for "prostate cancer" on CompuServe, Prodigy, and the Internet. The Prostate Cancer InfoLink address is http://www.comed.com/prostate/.

Case Histories: The Benefit of Support Groups

Robert J. was diagnosed with metastatic prostate cancer in his early sixties. He underwent severe emotional turmoil, including a serious depression, before hormonal therapy. The therapy put his cancer into almost complete remission. Based on this experience, Robert has dedicated himself to helping others through active leadership of a support group in New England. He is now in his third year of running the group, which is one of the most active and innovative in its outreach programs in this area. Robert has experienced a great catharsis by helping provide critical information to his fellow prostate cancer patients. This information includes detailed descriptions of treatment options as well as testimonials from men who have been treated by local clinicians.

"A lot of this information may come too late for me," Robert concedes. "But helping others make the best choices gives me great satisfaction."

James T. has recently been diagnosed with apparently localized prostate cancer. He was 60 years old when he underwent screening. His PSA level of 6.0 ng/ml but no abnormality on his DRE led to a biopsy, which produced a Gleason score of 6.

James was fearful of surgery because he'd heard the scuttlebutt at his office: "You'll spend the rest of your life impotent, wearing a diaper."

Although the doctors he consulted assured him that if side effects did occur they could be readily treated, James concedes that he felt they were overselling radical prostatectomy by downplaying the side effects. He attended a prostate cancer support group meeting, in which he was able to discuss his situation in great detail with men who had stood in his shoes before him.

"What I learned at those meetings," James later explained, "was that the side effects were much less severe than I'd been led to believe by the guys at work." He was relieved to learn that the mild incontinence several postsurgery patients had experienced was easily managed, tolerable, and would possibly disappear in time.

James has now undergone surgery. His tumor appears to have been completely organ confined. He is coping with sexual dysfunction and relatively minor incontinence.

*   *   *

The case histories presented in this book epitomize the experience of tens of thousands of American men over the past few years. For many of these men, PSA screening marked the beginning of a complicated medical odyssey. On this voyage, they had to face their own mortality and literally make life-and-death decisions about treatment. For several of these men, the treatments appear to have cured their prostate cancer.

You may be in the position they were in when they were screened. What you should learn from their experiences is that knowledge is crucial to making good decisions.

Were their decisions "right"? Most of them feel they took the correct course of action.

Would their choices meet your needs? That is a question that only you, your loved ones, and the medical team you seek for advice and treatment can adequately answer.

Nobody likes to make hard decisions. And it is only human to hate a dilemma. However, prostate cancer forces us to make difficult decisions and to confront unyielding dilemmas as we choose our best course among the pitfalls and obstacles of screening, diagnosis, and treatment. If we opt for screening and it leads to a diagnosis of prostate cancer, we must weigh the benefits of treatment against the probable risks of side effects.

Above all, prostate cancer is a disease replete with uncertainty. And this painful ambiguity often hits us at a time in our lives when we seek serenity. In my practice, I often meet men who are very angry that the tranquillity of later life has been so unfairly disrupted by the threat of prostate cancer.

In later life, we should have the strength and the knowledge to make decisions that are appropriate for us and our families. To do so, we need as much information as possible about an often unpredictable adversary. I hope that this book has provided you some of that critical information.

Glossary

Acid phosphatase An enzyme produced in the prostate. Before the advent of the prostate specific antigen assay, acid phosphatase tests were used to detect prostate disorders, including prostate cancer. It is not a good screening test for prostate cancer. Today this test is sometimes used in conjunction with the PSA to help determine if a cancer is likely to be cured with surgery.

Adrenal androgens Male hormones produced in the adrenal glands, which make up a small percentage of the circulating androgens affecting prostatic tissue. The majority of the androgens in the blood are from the testes.

Adrenal glands Glands located adjacent to each kidney that produce a variety of hormones, including male hormones called adrenal androgens.

Age-adjusted PSA value The concept of adjusting "normal" prostate-specific antigen levels by age to take into account the almost universal enlargement of the prostate with aging.

Agonist (also called analogs) Chemical mimics of certain compounds, including LH-RH agonists (analogs) such as leuprolide (Lupron) and gosereline (Zoladex). These agonists signal the pituitary to stop producing luteinizing hormone (LH) and thus decrease testosterone production. They are used as hormonal therapy for metastatic prostate cancer.

Analgesic A class of pain-relieving medications that ranges from over-the-counter drugs to narcotic analgesics.

Androgens Omnibus term for male hormones produced primarily in the testes and adrenal glands. Prostatic tissue is androgen dependent for metabolism and growth.

Antiandrogen   A medication that blocks the effect of male hormones.

Antiangiogenesis   A concept in oncology wherein tumors are deprived of new blood vessels (capillaries).

Artificial urethral sphincter   A surgically implanted prosthetic device used to control severe urinary incontinence.

Benign   The medical term for noncancerous tissue growth.

Benign prostatic hyperplasia (BPH)   The nonmalignant (benign) overgrowth of prostatic tissue, especially the stromal component. BPH occurs in many men as they age and can cause urinary symptoms related to blockage of urine flow, including frequent urination and decreased stream of urination.

Bicalutamide   An antiandrogen. Its brand name is Casodex.

Biopsy   The removal of tissue samples for pathologic examination to aid in diagnosis.

Biopsy of the prostate   A procedure that is most often performed transrectally, using a spring-loaded biopsy gun guided by an ultrasonic probe. Sextant biopsies (six samples) spanning the prostate's symmetric sides are usually obtained.

Bladder (urinary)   A muscular pouch in the lower abdomen that serves as the urinary reservoir; it is connected to the urethra (the urinary tube within the penis) and connected to the kidneys by the ureters.

Bone scan ("scintiscan" or "radioneuclide scintigraphy")   A diagnostic procedure in which radioisotopes are injected into the bloodstream and absorbed by bone. This is used to detect bone abnormalities, including prostate cancer metastases.

Cancer   The unnatural overgrowth of abnormal tissue that begins with genetic abnormality at the cellular level. Cancerous tumors are said to be "malignant": they invade normal tissue and have the ability to metastasize or spread malignant seeds elsewhere in the body.

Carcinoma   The form of cancer arising in the epithelial cells that form the lining of many structures, such as glands.

Catheter   A flexible tube that is often used in surgery to drain or irrigate body cavities. The Foley catheter is used to drain the urinary bladder during the healing process following prostate surgery.

Chemotherapy   Cancer treatment that involves medications that directly kill cells. Chemotherapy is meant to selectively kill malignant tumor cells. Drugs are commercially available to treat a variety of cancers.

Clinical stage   A term that describes the physicians' estimate of the extent of a malignant tumor. In prostate cancer, the clinical stage is estimated following a digital rectal examination and a bone scan.

Co-morbidity   Illnesses unrelated in any way to the cancer or treatment of the cancer that may compromise quantity or quality of life.

Corpora cavernosa   The paired erectile bodies in the dorsal (upper) area of the penis.

Computerized tomography   The CT scan, or CAT scan, is a computer-enhanced imaging tool that takes horizontal X-ray images of the body. CT scans produce much clearer images of soft tissue than do standard X-rays.

Deoxyribonucleic acid (DNA)   A molecule that comes in four different types. When strung together in different combinations, as in a chain, it can carry the genetic information in the nucleus of a cell.

Differentiation, cellular   A diagnostic concept that is assessed by the pathologist when he or she examines the malignant tissue. Well-differentiated cells of similar size and shape with distinct borders and nuclei are the least malignant. Poorly differentiated cells have heterogeneous size and bizarre shapes with poorly defined margins and abnormal nuclei.

Digital rectal examination (DRE)   A diagnostic procedure in which a physician palpates the prostate using a gloved finger inserted into the rectum. Physicians are trained to detect by touch hard nodules and abnormal enlargement of the gland that may indicate cancer.

Early prostate cancer   The disease stage at which a bone scan or CT scan have shown there to be no evidence of metastatic spread. At this stage, prostate cancer is considered potentially curable by surgery or radiation therapy.

Ejaculate   The fluid expelled from the penis during ejaculation. The testes, the seminal vesicles, and the prostate contribute material to the ejaculate.

Epididymis   The densely coiled structures at the top of each testicle where spermatozoa mature and are stored until ejaculation.

Epithelial tissue   A distinct class of cells that form the lining of anatomical structures and make up the functioning component of most glands. Prostate cancer arises in the epithelial, or glandular, component.

External-beam radiation therapy   Curative — A treatment involving high-energy X-ray radiation focused on the prostate and designed to kill malignant cancer cells within the gland. The principal side effects are sexual dysfunction and change in bowel function.
Palliative — A similar, but briefer duration use of high-energy X-rays to irradiate prostate cancer metastases, generally in bone.

Extracapsular prostate cancer   See *Early prostate cancer.* Descriptive stage of the disease in which cancer has penetrated through the capsule of the prostate and exists outside the gland. The disease may or may not be curable at this stage.

Finasteride (Proscar)   A drug in the class of 5-alpha reductase inhibitors that blocks the conversion of testosterone into dihydrotestosterone by prostate tissue. Finasteride is now used as a treatment for benign prostatic hyperplasia (BPH) and is being tested in conjunction with the antiandrogen flutamide as an alternative to standard hormonal therapy for metastatic prostate cancer.

Flow cytometry   A test performed on cancerous cells to determine the degree of DNA abnormality; it may correlate with the aggressiveness of the tumor.

Flutamide   An antiandrogen. Its brand name is Eulexin.

Gleason score (grading system)   The numerical system used to assess tumor differentiation. The scale is from 1 to 5, wherein 1 is well differentiated and 5 is poorly differentiated. The score is obtained by adding the grade numbers of the two most prominent types of malignant architecture from a tissue sample that is microscopically examined by a pathologist.

Hormone (or hormonal) therapy   The principal treatment for metastatic prostate cancer. This involves the ablation or deprivation of androgens (male hormones) so that malignant prostate cancer cells that are hormonally dependent will die and/or not reproduce. The principal forms of hormonal therapy are orchiectomy (surgical castration) or LH-RH agonist therapy.

Incontinence   Difficulty or inability to retain urine. Stress incontinence sometimes occurs following prostate cancer surgery (radical prostatectomy).

Laparoscopy   A technique used to perform surgery in which a fiber-optic device is used to visualize internal structures, and the surgery is performed through instruments, which gain access to the site of surgery through small skin incisions. Surgery is performed without surgical incisions on the abdomen. Lymph node removal for biopsy is now sometimes performed with this technique.

Luteinizing hormone (LH)   A chemical messenger produced by the pituitary gland that signals the production of the male hormone testosterone by the testes.

Luteinizing hormone-releasing hormone (LH-RH)   A brain hormone that signals the pituitary gland, causing it to produce luteinizing hormone (LH).

Lymphadenectomy   The surgical removal of lymph nodes. Lymphadenectomy is usually performed during the radical prostatectomy procedure but immediately before removal of the prostate so that pathologic examination can be conducted prior to prostate removal. Alternatively, lymphadenectomy is sometimes performed as a separate procedure (see *Laparoscopy*).

Magnetic resonance imaging (MRI)   A scanning technology that produces a clear image of body sections, including both bone and soft tissue. It is sometimes used to assess the extent of a prostate tumor using a device called an endorectal coil.

Margins, surgical   The dissected edge of surgically removed tissue. Pathologists examine these margins to determine if they are free of malignancy. If cancer has extended to the margins, it is probable that the disease has extended or spread beyond the original site.

Metastasis   A "seed" or small portion of a malignant tumor that has become established away from the primary site; the spread or extension of malignancy from a primary tumor to nearby or distant sites. Several metastatic sites are called metastases. These metastases frequently take months, and more likely years, before they can be seen on a scan.

Metastatic prostate cancer   Stage D disease in which the primary prostate tumor has spread or metastatized to structures beyond the gland, usually either the pelvic lymph nodes and/or the bone.

Morbidity   A medical term referring to the symptoms or the alteration in the quality of a person's life caused by a disease or its treatment.

Neurovascular bundle   Delicate structures of nerves and blood vessels that control penile erection. Neurovascular bundles adhere to the sides of the prostate. They are often removed with the gland during radical prostatectomy, causing postsurgical sexual dysfunction.

Observation   See *Watchful waiting.*

Orchiectomy (bilateral)   The surgical removal of both testes in order to reduce the level of circulating male hormones.

Organ-confined prostate cancer   Stage A or B in the Whitmore-Jewett staging system (T1a through T2c in the TNM system). The malignant tumor is confined to one or both sides of the prostate gland.

Palliative therapy   Noncurative treatment meant to relieve symptoms as part of an overall strategy to improve quality of life.

Perineum   The structure at the base of the pelvic cavity between the scrotum and the anus.

Prostate   An accessory sex gland in the human male that surrounds the urethra at the base of the urinary bladder. In the adult, the prostate weighs about 20 grams and has a spheroid shape approximately 1.6 inches in diameter; as a man ages, the prostate naturally grows in both weight and size. The prostate, which produces an important component of the seminal fluid, is composed of both stromal (connective) and epithelial (glandular) tissue.

Prostate-specific antigen (PSA)   A protein (enzyme) that is produced exclusively by prostate epithelial cells. PSA circulating in the blood stream can be detected and is generally measured in nanograms per milliliter of serum, ng/ml.

Prostate-specific antigen assay (PSA assay)   The standard blood test to detect and measure PSA levels in the blood.

Prostatic intra-epithelial neoplasia (PIN)   Abnormal glandular cells that a pathologist can recognize microscopically and which many clinicians believe is the precursor to prostate cancer.

Prostatism   Symptoms of BPH, including urinary frequency, hesitance, diminished force of stream, and frequent urination during the night.

PSA density   The level of PSA in ng/ml circulating in the blood divided by the estimated volume of the prostate gland.

PSA velocity   The rate of increase or decrease in PSA level during periodic PSA assays.

Radical prostatectomy   The curative surgical procedure during which the prostate, seminal vesicles, and a sampling of pelvic lymph nodes are removed. The most common procedure involves the retropubic surgical approach through the abdomen. The perineal surgical approach between the scrotum and the anus is less commonly used. Generally curative in the case of organ-confined prostate cancer, the principal side effects of the radical prostatectomy are sexual dysfunction and stress urinary incontinence.

Radiopharmaceuticals   Radioactive isotopes used in palliative therapy for metastatic prostate cancer. The principal radiopharmaceutical currently used is strontium-89, which is preferentially absorbed by bone and relieves the symptoms of bony metastases.

RT-PCR for PSA   Reverse-transcriptase polymerase chain reaction for prostate-specific antigen (PSA) test. New test capable of identifying prostate cancer cells in the blood, bone marrow, or lymph nodes. Although it is a very sensitive test, its value is still to be ascertained.

Scrotum   The fleshy pouch containing the testes and epididymis from which the vasa deferentia transport sperm during ejaculation.

Semen (ejaculate)   The viscous fluid expelled from the penis during ejaculation, which contains spermatozoa as well as nutrient and transport secretions from the prostate and seminal vesicles.

Seminal vesicle(s)   Paired glands with a leaf shape adjacent to the prostate beneath the lower posterior aspect of the bladder. Fluid from the seminal vesicles combines with spermatozoa and prostatic fluid during ejaculation. Involvement of the seminal vesicles with prostate cancer is seen by many as strong evidence for the potential of metastatic cancer.

Sign   Outward evidence of an illness or condition apparent to the patient and/or physician.

Staging of prostate cancer   Any of several clinical or pathological tests and procedures conducted to find the extent of disease. The two principal staging systems are the traditional Whitmore-Jewett system (stage A through D) and the more recent Tumor Nodes Metastasis (TNM) system (stage T1a through M+).

Stromal tissue   Muscular and connective tissue found throughout the prostate gland, which give the structure its shape and contract to expel prostatic fluid.

Symptom   A change in the way a patient feels or functions; a change in normal function, sensation, or appearance; a characteristic sign or indication of the existence of a disorder or disease.

Testosterone   The principal component of the male hormone circulating throughout the body. The ablation or deprivation of testosterone is the underpinning of hormonal therapy for metastatic prostate cancer.

Transurethral resection of the prostate (TURP)   The traditional surgical method of reducing BPH symptoms by excising benign tissue adjacent to the prostatic urethra. Today, medical therapy is more often used.

Ultrasonography   An imaging technique using ultrasonic waves to visualize internal tissues. The prostate is generally imaged by ultrasonography through a transrectal probe, a procedure that also guides transrectal prostate biopsy.

Urethra   The tube connecting the urinary bladder with the outside, which runs through the prostate and the penis.

Urethral sphincter   Also commonly called the external or striated urethral sphincter. The collarlike muscle group within the urethra below the prostate which constricts the urethra through voluntary and involuntary input to control the flow of urine.

Vas deferens   One of the paired fibrous tubes connecting the epididymis in the scrotum with the ejaculatory duct in the prostatic urethra, through which spermatozoa pass.

Watchful waiting (observation)   A strategy in which a patient diagnosed with prostate cancer is monitored without treatment. Generally, watchful waiting is used in older patients with limited life expectancy, those with apparently localized disease who do not want to endure the side effects of treatment, or those who are believed to have cancers that are not likely to be life threatening.

Appendix 1

Side Effects of Therapy: Radical Prostatectomy and External-Beam Radiation

Sexual Function

Symptom	Therapy	Pretherapy	Percentage with Symptoms	
			3 months	12 months
No erections in 4 weeks	RP[a]	11	85	75
	XRT[b]	18	25	33
Erections adequate for intercourse	RP[a]	32	96	93
	XRT[b]	45	58	67

[a] Radical prostatectomy
[b] External-beam radiation therapy

Based on Talcott et al.

Appendix 2

Side Effects of Therapy: Radical Prostatectomy and External-Beam Radiation

Urinary Incontinence

Symptom	Therapy	Pretherapy	Percentage with Symptoms	
			3 months	12 months
Wore pad in underwear	RP[a]	3	58	35
within last week	XRT[b]	1	5	5
Dribble urine	RP[a]	2	24	11
(moderate)	XRT[b]	1	2	2

[a] Radical prostatectomy
[b] External-beam radiation therapy

Based on Talcott et al.

Notes

2. Prostate Cancer in America Today

1. Another interesting finding is that certain hormones may protect against prostate cancer. The hormone dehydroepiandrosterone (DHEA) protects against the development of prostate cancer in rats. This compound certainly warrants closer study in people as a chemopreventive drug.

3. What Is Prostate Cancer?

1. Prostate cancer is one of a variety of different types of human carcinomas. These are malignant growths that arise in epithelial tissues: the skin, the lining of the digestive tract and blood vessels, and the internal organs, such as the pancreas, liver, ovaries, and the prostate gland. An important subcategory of carcinomas into which prostate cancer falls is called adenocarcinomas, "adeno" meaning glandlike. These are malignant tumors that grow in the glandular tissue of organs (the portion of the organ's structure that produces secretions). Some adenocarcinomas such as cancers of the pancreas and lung are almost always dangerously aggressive. Prostate cancer, though heterogeneous in its natural history, tends to be less aggressive than these other types of adenocarcinomas.

2. The most reliable standard for defining a growth as being cancerous is through pathology: the examination (most often microscopic) of a biopsy sample by a trained pathologist. A diagnosis of cancer can be made in certain cases at the level of molecular biology by identifying specific changes in the DNA of a cell's genes. Such genetic analyses are

being used more frequently these days and will undoubtedly be employed more widely in the future. This means that a much earlier diagnosis of cancer in growths we now call precancerous will be possible.

3. One of the most intensive areas of medical research in the last thirty years has been identifying the differences between cancerous cells and normal cells. For example, how do aggressive cancerous cells in the liver or pancreas differ from the normal tissue cells from which they arose? We often don't know which of the many differences between cancerous and normal cells are fundamental to the process of malignancy and which are of secondary importance.

5. Screening for Prostate Cancer

1. This was the conclusion of the 1991 research study published by Dr. William Catalona and colleagues in the *New England Journal of Medicine,* as well as several other studies.

2. The American Cancer Society's recommendation is: "Prostate exam" (DRE and PSA) for men fifty and over, every year. The ACS does not formally recommend an age to cease screening.

The recommendation of the American Urological Association for "early detection of prostate cancer" is:

"Annual digital rectal examination (DRE) and serum prostate specific antigen (PSA) measurement substantially increase the early detection of prostate cancer. These tests are most appropriate for male patients 50 years of age or older and for those 40 or older who are at high risk, including those of African-American descent and those with a family history of prostate cancer. Patients in these age/risk groups should be given information about these tests and should be given the option to participate in screening or early detection programs. PSA testing should continue in a healthy male who has a life expectancy of ten years or more.

"PSA and DRE are used for the early detection of prostate cancer. The use of prostate ultrasound is best reserved to evaluate those patients who have an abnormal digital rectal examination and/or abnormal PSA level.

"Transrectal prostate ultrasonography can be used as an adjunctive procedure for the diagnosis of prostate cancer. Prostate ultrasonography serves as a method of determining prostate volume, and sonographic guidance can enhance the accuracy of prostate biopsy, particularly of small lesions."

3. The only way to prove that PSA screening for prostate cancer significantly reduces the number of men who die of the disease would be to conduct what we call a randomized, prospective research study, which has not yet been carried out on a large scale. Randomized studies are those in which the treatment, the test, or the intervention being studied is assigned to an individual randomly, usually through a computer-generated selection method. Thus, in the case of a randomized study of prostate cancer screening, about half the people would be screened and half would not.

Research studies under way might not yield results for another ten or fifteen years. If you're a middle-aged man, this research won't benefit you. You've got to make decisions *now* that might affect the rest of your life, so you must make those decisions based on other factors.

4. The Canadian counterpart of the task force is officially opposed to using the PSA to test men without symptoms. The National Cancer Institute has remained neutral on the issue of PSA testing.

Ann Flood, a public health policy expert at Dartmouth College's Center for Evaluation of Clinical Sciences, summarized the controversy: "What's fascinating is that really informed deliberative bodies have come up with diametrically opposed conclusions."

The Congressional Office of Technology Assessment released a report in May 1995 that concluded, "Research has not yet been completed to determine whether systematic, early screening for prostate cancer extends lives."

5. It is worth noting that this issue is so vexing that medical researchers have been working on decision analyses to determine if prostate cancer screening is beneficial. Using research data on clinical outcomes of screening and treatment, researchers are trying to determine the likelihood of benefit of different options: no screening; screening followed by surgery; screening followed by radiation therapy; screening followed by watchful waiting. One such decision-analysis model found no clear benefits in screening for prostate cancer. This study has been criticized for its use of allegedly biased data, however.

6. An FDA announcement cited the "many questions" that still re-

main within the medical community about the best way to screen for, diagnose, and treat prostate cancer.

6. Treatment of Early Prostate Cancer I

1. The normal serum PSA test measures the protein secreted into the blood. Using sophisticated molecular techniques, it is also possible to detect very low abundance ribonucleic acid (RNA) unique to specific types of cells. Using RT-PCR, we can discern RNA unique to prostate epithelial cells. This test can detect one PSA-producing cell among 10^6 or 10^7 RNA-producing cells. Therefore, it is possible to detect cells that produce this RNA, even if there are only small numbers of such cells circulating in the blood.

Normally, prostate cells are confined to the gland, but they can spread beyond the gland if a prostate cancer has more aggressive character-istics. Researchers at a number of institutions, including the Dana-Far-ber Cancer Institute, explored the idea that prostate cancer patients may have malignant prostate cells circulating in their blood that could be detected by RT-PCR. The test is so sensitive that even a few prostate cells could be discerned in a blood sample by identifying its unique RNA.

As anticipated, patients free of prostate cancer did not have cells circulating in their blood producing this specific RNA. But the research also proved that men with prostate cancer did have circulating prostate cells that could be detected by the RT-PCR assay.

Men with localized prostate cancer, however, had detectable circulat-ing cells less frequently than men with metastatic disease. This finding was to be expected, as, in metastatic prostate cancer, there is a much higher probability of circulating cells.

Recently published studies reveal an interesting aspect of this RT-PCR research. Researchers at Columbia Presbyterian studied men un-dergoing radical prostatectomy who were diagnosed with localized dis-ease before surgery. A portion of these men had cancer that had spread beyond the capsule of the gland, either into seminal vesicles, or to the surgical margins when the pathologist examined the entire prostate following removal. A significant number of these men also tested posi-tive on the RT-PCR assay.

This suggested that patients with localized cancer who test positive on the RT-PCR assay had a lower likelihood of being cured by surgery.

The authors suggested that such patients should avoid surgery. These findings are very provocative but must be considered preliminary and need to be substantiated by large-scale studies before any treatment policy is derived from them.

2. Researchers at Johns Hopkins University studied patients with stage T1C cancers (cancers detected by elevated PSA alone that prompted a biopsy) and who then underwent radical prostatectomy. Patients who had only one positive biopsy core and low PSA densities had cancers that were extremely low-volume and low-grade at the time of surgery. Such cancers may have a low metastatic potential. In other words, these tumors are reasonably good candidates for the category of prostate cancers that remain relatively dormant, confined to the gland throughout the remaining years of the man's life, even if he receives no treatment at all. These data need to be confirmed.

3. Some oncologists believe that there should be a major distinction for cancers that have any component of Gleason 4. This could be, for example, a grade 4 over 3. Thus a Gleason score 7 could have some grade 4 component and behave significantly more aggressively than a Gleason 6. These subtle distinctions need further clarification. At the moment it is difficult to make clinical decisions based on these differences.

4. Cancers that have grossly abnormal numbers of chromosomes on a per-cell basis tend to behave more aggressively. A technique called flow cytometry, which assesses the DNA ploidy (the number of copies of DNA that the average cell contains), may add more information about aggressive potential than that obtained from the grading system alone.

7. Treatment of Early Prostate Cancer II

1. Most urologists conducting a radical prostatectomy remove a representative sampling of pelvic lymph nodes early in the procedure (before the surgical dissection of the prostate) for immediate pathological examination. If the pathologist detects cancer in the pelvic lymph nodes — stage D1 (N+) at the time of surgery — most urologists will not perform the radical prostatectomy and instead close the incision. The fundamental therapeutic purpose of the radical prostatectomy is to remove the prostate before the cancer has spread beyond the confines of the gland.

Other urologists, however, believe it is important to remove the gland, which is the primary tumor site, even though the cancer has spread to the pelvic lymph nodes. This is certainly an aggressive treatment approach, but one which is of uncertain value.

As to the course of action following the detection of positive lymph nodes, I do not see any utility in continuing the radical prostatectomy if these nodes contain cancer cells. This is evidence that malignant cells have spread outside the gland. And, if these tiny malignant seeds have already spread to other parts of the body, surgical removal of the prostate — with all of the side effects this entails — will not appreciably, if at all, alter this condition.

2. Patrick Walsh's radical prostatectomy is clearly a marked improvement in technique. Even if surgeons are reluctant to leave the neurovascular bundles intact, they work with much greater precision than in the past. This means that surgeons can cut a lower margin near the external urethral sphincter but not damage the cylindrical collar of striated muscle that controls urine flow. Also, it is now much easier to remove the two seminal vesicles from the posterior fascia (connective tissue) between the lower bladder and the rectum without fear of damaging either of these structures. In short, the Walsh procedure makes the operation safer and definitely reduces postsurgical side effects, even if sexual function is altered.

3. We may see the RT-PCR for PSA technique applied to the detection of cancer in lymph nodes since this is a much more sensitive test for cancer cells than just looking for the cells under the microscope. In a very preliminary study conducted by Dr. Robert Edelstein and colleagues, patients who were positive in an RT-PCR for PSA text had a higher likelihood of relapse after radical prostatectomy than did those patients who were negative. These results need to be confirmed.

4. We have studied this problem closely at Dana-Farber. Dr. James Talcott asked 125 patients about urine control prior to surgery as well as three months and twelve months after surgery performed by a variety of surgeons from different hospitals. It was unusual for men to have complete urinary incontinence soon after radical prostatectomy, although it did occur. Many men needed the added protection of a pad to protect against incontinence for weeks or months after the surgery was performed. The most important fact was that, a year after surgery, over 30 percent of postoperative patients still used some reinforcement.

But it is unclear why incontinence happens in some men and not others (see Appendix 2).

5. There has been controversy about the true benefits of the nerve-sparing procedure. Many surgeons using Dr. Walsh's procedure have not been able to duplicate his results.

Dr. James Talcott of Dana-Farber also studied sexual function in men after radical prostatectomy. Our study looked at the effect of radical prostatectomy on men who averaged 62 years old. Most of them were sexually potent prior to surgery. But one year after the surgery, almost 80 percent of the men were unable to achieve erections normally. And the small percentage who could do so were unable to achieve an erection adequate for intercourse.

Many of the men we studied had undergone the nerve-sparing radical prostatectomy procedure. Based on our research, we and a growing group of others feel that the results of the nerve-sparing procedure in maintaining sexual function have been greatly overstated. This is probably because the factors in the procedure that compromise sexual function go beyond merely sparing the nerves.

8. Treatment of Early Prostate Cancer III

1. Without randomized studies, prospective research is the next most valuable line of investigation. This involves collecting baseline information from patients and following their clinical progress over time. However, data of this sort is minimal for prostate cancer.

2. The studies to date comparing tumor volume and metastatic potential were conducted on a small number of prostatectomy specimens. Large-population, randomized studies that can produce statistically significant findings are needed.

3. The best available research findings on watchful waiting (observation) or deferred therapy come from a paper by Dr. Gerald Chodak and others, published in the *New England Journal of Medicine,* in which they pooled the results of six studies available in the medical literature. These studies covered 828 patients of a variety of ages and diverse tumor characteristics. All these patients were followed for a minimum of ten years without initial therapy.

Thirteen percent of the patients with low-grade tumors had died by the end of the ten-year observation period.

Thirteen percent of the patients with intermediate-grade tumors had died by the end of the ten-year observation period.

Sixty-six percent of the patients with high-grade tumors had died by the end of the ten-year observation period.

4. These studies indicate that most cancers being detected by present PSA-screening methods look like clinically significant tumors. The average volume and pathological grade of these tumors are those that most clinicians would treat. But it remains to be seen whether sequential screening — in which large numbers of patients undergo periodic PSA tests — will produce widespread evidence of clinically significant cancers throughout the population. I suspect that, as the screening net is cast farther, the cancers detected will begin to appear less aggressive; there will probably be higher proportions of smaller, lower-grade tumors. And the proportion of cancers that are clinically insignificant will increase.

9. Life after Treatment

1. The side effect of sexual dysfunction is common following both radical prostatectomy and radiation therapy. Research conducted at our institution indicates that one year after treatment, almost 80 percent of postprostatectomy patients who had surgery at a variety of hospitals and who were potent prior to surgery were impotent after surgery, compared to over 40 percent of postradiation patients. Moreover, in these studies, only 7 percent of postprostatectomy patients were able to achieve an erection adequate for sexual intercourse. This compares to 33 percent of postradiation patients who achieved erections adequate for sexual intercourse one year after treatment (see Appendix 1). After two years the rates of sexual dysfunction from external-beam radiation approach those of radical prostatectomy. Thus it is probably unwise to select external-beam radiation over surgery in the hope that it will preserve sexual function; it seems to just take longer for dysfunction to occur.

10. Metastatic Prostate Cancer I: Hormonal Therapy

1. LH-RH analogs (or blockers) are chemical mimics of the naturally occurring hormone LH-RH. LH-RH is released by the hypothalamus of the lower brain and signals the pituitary gland to release luteinizing

hormone (LH). LH-RH blockers are similar in structure to LH-RH but act by preventing the LH-RH signal from reaching your pituitary gland. The ultimate result is the almost complete cessation of testicular androgen production.

2. John Brukovsky from Vancouver has produced evidence that the emergence of androgen-independent tumor cells indeed depends on the total androgen milieu in your body. Androgen-independent cells may emerge and reproduce more rapidly in the setting of androgen deprivation during hormonal therapy, even though these clones have no metabolic dependence on androgens. He suggests that the length of remission after hormonal therapy is probably a function of the proportion of androgen-dependent to androgen-insensitive cell clones in the original tumor.

This provides the experimental basis for intermittent suppression or ablation of androgens. In this approach, your physician generates androgen deprivation by medical intervention (LH-RH analogs) and then withdraws the therapy to allow your androgen milieu to regenerate. After testosterone production rises again, your levels return to near-normal, the androgen ablation therapy is resumed. Intermittent hormonal therapy — interrupting LH-RH treatment — theoretically delays the proliferation of insensitive clones. This interesting concept has shown promise in animal studies but is unproven in human research.

12. Metastatic Prostate Cancer III: Systemic and Experimental Treatment of the Cancer

1. These drugs are sometimes used in conjunction with low doses of steroids to supplement the non-androgen steroid production from the adrenal glands. Steroids can also have anticancer activity in their own right. Interestingly, ketoconazole was originally developed as an antifungal drug but was found to have activity in prostate cancer. In some advanced prostate cancer patients, a course of ketoconazole may cause the cancer to go into remission. And, if ketoconazole or aminoglutethimide lowers a patient's PSA, this is an indication that there is still a significant proportion of hormonally sensitive malignant cells present.

2. There are some malignancies, such as testicular cancer, Hodgkin's disease, and non-Hodgkin's lymphoma, that are far more sensitive to chemotherapy. Breast cancer cells are also sensitive to some forms of chemotherapy. However, oncologists understand that chemotherapy

usually does not kill every metastatic breast cancer cell in a person's body. The treatment can bring remission, but actual cure is rare.

3. There is a small subset of patients whose metastatic prostate cancer takes an unusual form, called neuroendocrine-type or small-cell carcinoma. These malignant cells appear microscopically to be similar to some cancers that affect the lung. If a patient's prostate cancer acquire this form, they are sensitive to certain types of chemotherapy. Only a small percentage of advanced prostate cancer patients, however, fall into this category.

4. Suramin presumably controls cellular reproduction by diverting chemical growth factors needed for mitosis.

5. Other research targets include the ability of tumors to gain access to the blood supply (degrading enzymes called proteinases) or metastasize. Drugs are being developed that interfere with these processes. Some are now in clinical trials.

6. Research has shown that interleukin-2 has the potential to fortify the immune system and thus may help to destroy malignant cells throughout the body.

Doctors first extracted T cells from the circulating blood of patients with advanced malignant melanoma, which is almost always fatal. These T cells were grown outside the body with interleukin-2, then injected back into the patients. Thus activated, the so-called lymphokine activated killer cells targeted the melanoma metastases. In 1986, Steven Rosenberg and colleagues announced that about a quarter of the patients treated showed dramatic tumor shrinkage. Clearly, this approach has been very promising.

Rosenberg's research team extracted T cells called tumor-infiltrating lymphocytes directly from primary tumors and metastases. This was a logical step, because the immune-system cells obviously arose in response to the presence of malignant tissue but were simply not strong enough or lacked some critical factor to destroy all the cancer cells. When infused with interleukin-2 and reinjected in the patient, these T cells appeared to be active in some tumors.

More recently, researchers have attempted to enhance the tumor-infiltrating lymphocytes' ability to kill cancer cells by adding a gene that expresses a naturally occurring immune system substance, including tumor necrosis factor, or IL-2.

To date, this immunotherapy approach has been tested against a variety of cancers with only modest results.

Acknowledgments

I am deeply indebted to my mentors, George Canellos, M.D., and Robert Mayer, M.D., for their mentorship early in my career; to my colleagues, C. Norman Coleman, M.D., Edward Moss, M.D., Jerome Richie, M.D., and James Talcott, M.D., for helping me formulate my approach to this disease; to Claire Beard, M.D., Stephen Brecher, Ph.D., Anthony D'Amico, M.D., Ph.D., Lawrence Halpern, Cathy Hogan, R.N., A.O.C.N., Richard Howe, Ph.D., Irving Kaplan, M.D., Patricia Rieker Ph.D., William Whitmore and Kenneth Wishnow, M.D., for critical review of the manuscript; to Myles Brown, M.D., Margaret Bryant, R.N., Pamela Fontaine-Rothe, R.N., Kathleen Kenney, Kevin Loughlin, M.D., Richard Marlink, M.D., Francisco Trilla, M.D., and Anthony Zietman, M.D., for helpful discussion of all the issues involved with prostate cancer; and to Thomas Tisch, Joni Evans, and Alexandra Penny for making this book possible.

Index

experimental treatments, 191–
97
and quackery or questionable
treatment, 197–99
second-line hormonal therapy,
186–87
prognosis for, 143, 147–48
psychosocial support for, 200–
202
routes of spread of, 171–72
support groups on, 205–6
wives of patients with, 203–4
Metastron, 177
Milken, Michael, 197
Mitosis, 18
Molecular biology, 18, 19
Morbidity, 75, 96, 113, 213
Morphine, 174–75
MRI (magnetic resonance imaging), 27, 28, 69
and metastases, 145
and neurological impairment,
181
postsurgery, 129
and radiation implants, 101
and staging, 76
Mulligan, Richard, 196
Mutations, 11, 18–19
acquiring of, 116
and cancer, 19
in tumors, 166

National Cancer Institute, Information, 205
Natural history of cancer, 33, 36
of prostate cancer, 19, 33, 34–37
and age of patient, 10–11
and screening, 48, 49, 50
variability of, 33, 36, 73, 116
Neoadjuvant hormone therapy, 90–
91, 110

Neovasculature, 193
Nerve-sparing operation (radical
prostatectomy), 81–82, 86,
224n.2, 225n.5
Neuroendocrine-type cancers,
228n.3
Neurovascular bundle, 6, 81, 213–
14
Nizoral, 187
Nocturia, 8
Nonsteroidal anti-inflammatory
drugs (NSAIDs), 173, 175

Observation. See Watchful waiting
Oesterling, Joseph E., 44
Older men
and cure vs. quality of life, 110
and screening, 71, 122–23
See also Age
Orchiectomy, 108, 149, 153, 155,
214
with antiandrogens, 157–58
case history on, 156–57
side effects of, 156
Organ-confined prostate cancer,
79, 214
and surgery, 114
Pain, metastatic, 146, 169–71
and bone sites, 171–72
in case history, 157
and fractures, 178–79
and hormonal therapy, 150, 152,
155
and last stages, 182, 201
medications for, 172–75
from neurological impairment,
181
radiation therapy for, 170, 175–
77, 185
radiopharmaceuticals for, 177–
78